One Percent

My Journey Overcoming
Heart Disease

by
Thomas Martin
www.InOnePercent.com

This publication contains the opinion and ideas of the author. It is intended to provide helpful and informative material on the subjects addressed in the publication. It is sold with the understanding the author publisher are not engaged in rendering medical, health, or any other kind of personal professional services in the book. The reader should consult his or her medical, health, or other competent professional before adopting any of the suggestions in this book or drawing inference from it.

The author and publisher specifically disclaim all responsibility for any liability, loss, or risk, personal or otherwise, which is incurred as a consequence, directly or indirectly, of the use and application of any of the contents of this book.

Wasteland Press

www.wastelandpress.net
Shelbyville, KY USA

One Percent: My Journey Overcoming Hearth Disease
by Thomas Martin

First Printing – December 2011
ISBN: 978-1-60047-669-3

Printed in the U.S.A.

0   1   2   3   4   5   6

For Anna Bement and Sandy Coleman
To both I owe a debt I can never repay

Special Thanks

Dr. Peter Hoagland

Dr. Robert Adamson

Dr. David Brownstein

Dr. Mark Filidei

Dr. Mark Starr

Dr. Rodger Murphree

Kristi Ortiz

Leslie Hazard

Suzanne Chillcott

Marcia Stahovich

Sally Fallon

Dr. Kris Kennedy

Dr. Duane Graveline

Barbara Katzka

Kevin Chan

Wayne Lam

Mark Taylor

Dr. Richard Sacks

Ivon Visalli

Natasha Berechko

Haoi Nguyen

Richard Baker

Amy Tong

Delores Miron

Elizabeth Fitzgerald

Susan Richardson

Stephen Lizcano

Cindy Post

Michael, David, Peter & Sam Bement

Chris Bement

Jim and Mary Garlock

Ruth Sorenson

Bob and Peggy Sorenson

Pastor Melissa

Pastor Marc

Jennifer, Connor, Caroline & Calvin Veliz

Billie Ryan

Mona Davis

Rey & Marcris Cuevas

Jay Marzullo

Larry Trotter

Mark Taylor

Irena & Mike Medavoy

Richard Baker

Dr. Gregg Alzate

Natasha Berechko

Keith & Denise Rosier

A very special thanks to Roger & Kathy Massengale who firmly nudged me into writing this book.

Anissa, Dana, Lisa Gonzales, Lori, Laura, Enjoli, Pailai, Leah, Jason, Melissa, Sarah, Marcus, Mike Nibeker, Zan, Carol, Cindy, Elaine, Terry, Steve, James, Christina, Jen, Liz, Meagan, Esther, Dawn, Melissa, Emily, John, Sam and the entire nursing staff of 5 West and Surgical ICU. You are all the best!!

Table of Contents

Introduction

This book is about my physical decline from heart failure, my search for answers and the path I followed to overcome the disease.

In seeking answers, I read many, many books, something most people are unlikely to do. The need for answers also forced me to confront several of my doctors and challenge their approach to treating me. Sadly, this, too, is something most people are reluctant to do.

I originally thought of writing a book in which I would condense into one resource many of the findings from the books I had read. My problem with this is that I am not a doctor or a scientist. I am an engineer and, therefore, anything I write would not be based on my clinical experience; it would be based on the experiences of others. Instead, I decided to write my own story.

My objective in writing this book is not to provide all of the answers. It is more to point the reader in the direction that helped me. If you are serious about good health and wellness, you have a lot more work ahead of you. My book is also intended to make you question what you believe you already know.

As my health declined, I was fortunate to have people in my life who could point me toward resources and authors who might provide answers. This is something I know most people do not have. One question that came up repeatedly as I talked to people is, "Yes, but how do I know who to trust?" This is a very valid point, as you are likely to find books taking either side of any health issue. Which is right? Which is wrong?

I formed a baseline and what I read would have to meet these criteria for it to be something I would consider doing for myself. The first element of that baseline is: what is good for our bodies and what is not. Our bodies were either made or evolved eating organic, natural foods. Our grocery stores are now filled with genetically modified produce and foods designed purely for long shelf life or ease of preparation with little regard to its nutritional value.

If you add a pint of water to the gas tank of your car every time you fill up, you will, over time, destroy your engine. There is nothing wrong with water, but it is something your car engine is not designed to handle. The same is true for our bodies. If we keep feeding them garbage or continue ingesting synthetic drugs, we will not reach health, we will remain in a state of "dis-ease." Drugs are especially insidious. They are all synthetic and therefore all will have negative effects on our bodies over time. Is it any wonder that so many of the commercials on television are for drugs and so many others are for law firms suing drug companies?

Most of the chronic diseases we see can be traced back to deficiencies in our diets. But, "modern" medicine primarily treats symptoms and treats them using synthetic drugs. Neither approach solves the root problem, and they often make the problems worse.

For example, my cousin Anna's son, Peter, was only 8 years old when he began showing signs of malnutrition. Anna took him to his doctor only to be told, "He's fine, stop worrying about him." Peter would eat heartily, but continued losing weight, so much so that he began looking, as Anna described it, "like a holocaust victim." His stomach was distended, his eyes sunken, his skin was unusually pale, he would vomit after many meals; yet after repeated visits to the doctor, the doctor's evaluation never changed, "He's fine."

Then, Peter began sleepwalking, another sign that his body was starved for nutrition. Since no answers were coming from Peter's doctor and Anna was not going to sit by and watch her son die, she began searching for her own answers. As she read, everything kept pointing to Celiac disease. Celiac disease damages the wall of the small intestine and prevents proper absorption of nutrients. It is no wonder Peter was starving to death in spite of his healthy diet and appetite. Sufferers of Celiac cannot process gluten: a protein found in wheat, rye and barley. After learning this, Anna asked the doctor to test Peter for Celiac.

Her doctor refused, replying, "Peter definitely does not have Celiac."

Anna persisted and the doctor finally relented. Peter was tested and it was discovered he had Celiac disease. Anna put her entire family on a gluten-free diet and Peter responded immediately.

I include this story for the following three reasons:

- First, to point out the importance of taking control of your own health.
- Second, your doctor doesn't necessarily know everything nor have all the answers. In fact, your doctor can be flat out *wrong*.
- Third, the solution to Peter's problem was not in a drug, but in his diet.

I believe these same points are true for almost all ailments. It is the attitude I took when first diagnosed with heart failure. My attitude was that there was a reason and there was a solution. But, it was also up to me to find the answers and make the appropriate changes in my life to get well. I hope you, too, are ready to find the answers and take control of your own health.

Starting with our diets. We have been given so much misinformation over the years that it is no wonder we, as a society, have so many chronic diseases. For diet alone, I strongly recommend reading the book, "Nourishing Traditions" by Sally Fallon. It lays out an attitude and an approach to a healthy, traditional diet. I made many changes to my diet and to my preparation of foods. Also, I am fortunate to live in an area where there is a wide variety of markets catering to specialized food demands. So, I have ready access to such items as raw, whole milk.

We did not evolve nor were we created as vegans. Our eye-teeth show we are meat eaters and this is what our bodies still demand to function properly. Not only animal protein, but animal (saturated) fat as well.

If you would like to see pictures of my decline and recovery, please visit my website at www.InOnePercent.com.

Part I

My Journey

"Hope is a good thing, maybe the best of things."
- The Shawshank Redemption

September 2009

Thursday, September 17, 2009

At work, I walk the short distance to the cafeteria to get breakfast. Yet when I return to my desk, my breathing is short and shallow. What is wrong? I am only fifty years old; I have been in excellent health my entire life. I am tall, trim and have never smoked cigarettes. My only real vice is wine with dinner. I have never even been in a hospital, save as a child to have my tonsils removed. This can't be serious, I decide. I am confident the breathing difficulty will just go away on its own.

October 2009

Tuesday, October 6, 2009

Roughly twenty days later I fly to Portland, Oregon to celebrate my friend Cindy's birthday. We have a great day exploring the city. We drink cappuccino at a sidewalk café; we visit Powell's mega-emporium of used books and end the day in a trendy restaurant, eating ourselves into a state of ecstasy. We then drive the sixty minutes to her place in southern Washington. I feel as good as if I were a thirty-year-old man again, and I sleep well.

Wednesday, October 7, 2009

We spend the better part of the day hiking in a beautiful wooded area. The trees and sunlight are a symphony of light, dark and forest green. We lose our way, yet keep walking. We eventually need to find the car, but are in no hurry. We walk three or four miles before we stumble upon the correct route. We go home, have a light dinner; I begin to read "The Right Stuff," which I bought at Powell's, and by 9:30 p.m. I am ready to sleep. I drift off.

Thursday, October 8, 2009

I awake at 2:00 a.m. to a faint noise. I lie quietly in bed trying to determine the sound and its source. It is close to me but like nothing I have ever heard. I then realize it is emanating from inside my chest. It is a rale: an abnormal breathing sound. With each breath I exhale, the noise continues. I am concerned, but not panicked. Since I have no reference for serious illness, I simply assume all will be well.

But I am concerned enough to finally sit up, go to my computer and begin searching for answers. Pneumonia? Could that be it? I bring up a diagnostic website and begin reading about walking pneumonia. Yes, doubtless, that is the problem. I don't have all of the symptoms but it must be pneumonia. Nothing to be too concerned about. It is very treatable. I'll see a doctor, I decide, when I get back to California.

In spite of my brilliant diagnosis, something deep inside knows it is worse than I am willing to consider. What if I do have a serious problem? What then? These things do happen; I know this and I am somewhat frightened by the possibilities. Because of this, I cannot get back to sleep. I stay up the rest of the night reading my book, distracting myself with the adventures of Chuck Yeager and the Mercury astronauts.

Friday, October 9, 2009

I return home to Southern California with good memories of the Portland/Vancouver area and a persistent rale in my chest. A very odd pair of souvenirs.

Sunday, October 11, 2009

The noise does not go away and I begin feeling discomfort in my chest. I decide it is time to get checked at an urgent care center near my home. I explain my symptoms to the doctor as well as telling him my doubtlessly spot-on diagnosis.

He is somewhat skeptical. "Your symptoms are not fully consistent with pneumonia. I want a chest x-ray." When the doctor examines the x-ray, he seems to choose his words carefully. "I'm treating you for pneumonia but I also want you to see a cardiologist. It appears your heart is enlarged."

I selectively hear, "I'm treating you for pneumonia; if that doesn't work then maybe you need to see a cardiologist." I choose to ignore the part about the enlarged heart. Secretly, I hope this doctor flunked x-ray reading in medical school.

Saturday, October 17, 2009

Almost one week later I find myself parking my car centrally between where I plan to meet a friend for dinner and the theatre we'll be attending later. As I walk the three blocks to the restaurant, my breathing becomes labored and I feel pain in my chest. The rale continues even though I have been taking antibiotics for a week. I begin feeling panicky. I know something is seriously wrong, but I can't yet face up to it. After the theatre, I walk to my car with great difficulty as the pain keeps getting worse. It is as if someone with long, pointed fingernails is reaching into my lungs, grabbing and twisting them. I am not sure what to do, and I still cannot fully accept the severity of the situation.

I decide to call a friend of a friend, a doctor to see what she will say. I wake her with my call and in her fog she listens to my story and quietly and calmly asks questions as if she is not bothered at all by my late phone call. Not surprisingly, she does not provide me with a simple diagnosis. She suggests I drive to the emergency room for a full assessment.

I go home, go to bed and wait to see how I will feel in the morning.

Sunday, October 18, 2009

I take the day off and rest. I'm trying to believe that nothing serious is wrong with me, but I don't do an effective job. I am afraid and concerned and my body feels odd – like nothing I've ever felt before.

Monday, October 19, 2009

The pain and congestion in my chest does not ease. I return to urgent care for what I hope is a more optimistic opinion of my situation. I hope the doctor sees something he missed the first time. Something that does not include a problem with my heart. My hopes are not realized.

I see a different doctor than before and tell him I am still experiencing similar symptoms; but now I also feel pain in my chest.

He reads the prior doctor's notes and asks, "Have you seen a cardiologist?"

"No," I say with a sheepish grin on my face.

"Sit tight, I am calling a cardiologist right now to get you an appointment."

He exits the room, leaving me with my thoughts. I decide it is probably my turn to have a good health scare, but I also keep rationalizing that a scare is all it possibly can be.

When the doctor returns, he informs me, "You have an appointment tomorrow at 2:00 p.m."

Tuesday, October 20, 2009

Dr. Rita Bailey (not her real name), cardiologist, has her office in an open-air medical building. I park my car and begin wandering around, looking for her suite. I finally discover that it is on the second floor and I ascend the stairs. I enter her office and wait nervously.

Shortly, I am called to an examination room and meet with Dr. Bailey. She listens to my heart and lungs and decides to do my first of what will be many echocardiograms. I strip to the waist, lie on a table on my side and Dr. Bailey begins moving a wand across my chest, gathering information on my heart. She finishes, asks me to sit up and dress and she leaves the room. Sitting alone, I hope maybe she found nothing, that the doctors at the urgent care center were mistaken.

Dr. Rita Bailey marches back into my room, looks at me and growls, "You have heart failure. I can't even *believe* you were able to walk into my office unassisted. Just sit *right* where you are. I am calling another cardiologist and referring your case to him. He will probably put you in the hospital immediately!" She whirls and leaves the room.

Does this woman have a heart? A soul? I wonder. I am left with emotions I am not prepared to handle. She attacked me as if this is my fault, I think, as if I am in some way responsible. It isn't as if I am a heavy smoker or a diabetic; I have always been careful about my health.

Unsure of what to do, I pick up my cell phone, call my brother and begin to cry. Does this mean I'm dying? Is my time short? What do I do? "Heart failure" is a phrase that doesn't seem to be able to be manipulated into something that isn't extremely bad. I try controlling my sobs and tell him I need to see him; I need to talk to someone about this news.

He says he will drive down immediately and meet with me.

"Wait," I say, "let me find out what will happen next. I may end up in the hospital."

Dr Bailey returns to my room and tells me I have an appointment the next day with Dr. Michaels, a cardiologist who specializes in heart failure.

"Tomorrow?" I ask. "I thought you said this is serious."

She replies, "Apparently Dr Michaels doesn't see it quite that way, but he wants to see you soon."

I leave her office, pull myself together and call my brother again. I tell him not to come down; I am okay for now.

Wednesday, October 21, 2009

I ask my neighbor, Steve, to drive me to my appointment. I am not sure if I will be admitted to the hospital and would like to have a friend with me. I've never been in the hospital before and the enormity of what is happening is beginning to catch up with me.

Dr. Evan Michaels (not his real name) quietly enters the examination room and says little. He orders a wide array of blood tests, listens to my heart, squeezes my ankles and tells me he is scheduling me for an angiogram in two weeks. He hands me an order for the blood tests and leaves the room.

Based on his behavior, especially compared to Dr. Rita, I assume things can't be quite as bad as advertised. Of course I am wrong, but you know what they saying about assuming things.

I go downstairs to the lab and they draw multiple vials of blood.

I go home knowing little more than I did when I first entered the building. I am quite unhappy about how I am being treated. If I ever treated a client in this way in my career, I tell myself, I would have been fired. I guess different rules apply when one is wearing that white coat!

Monday, October 26, 2009

Five days later, I head back to Dr. Michaels' office. He goes through, what I will come to discover are his usual motions of listening to my heart, then my lungs and then pinching my ankles.

He finishes and says, "I'll see you next week for the angiogram."

I am stunned and upset!!

He then stands and turns to leave the room.

"Wait," I say, "what about the blood tests? What did you find?"

"Oh nothing, everything is fine," he replies.

What? Everything is *fine*? I have heart disease, heart failure, cardiomyopathy dilated. What do you mean, everything is fine?

"What is the reason for my heart failure?" I ask.

"We don't know," he says." We hope to learn more from the angiogram." And with that, he leaves the room.

My level of frustration with Dr. Michaels continues to rise. Why won't this man *talk* to me??? Tell me what he is thinking? Even if it is only an "educated guess." Hell, even *I* can do that!

November 2009

Monday, November 2, 2009

My cousin Sandy drives the seventy-five miles from her house to mine to take me for this morning's angiogram. Sandy is a nurse and wants to ensure that everyone takes good care of me. She and I used to spend summers together at our grandparents' house on the edge of nowhere in Needles, California. In such a God-forsaken place, you have nothing to do but bond. Now, she is here for me and she pretty much stays with me through the nightmare of the next nine months. Today is merely the first step.

I check into the hospital at 6:30 a.m. and am shown to my room. My nurse enters, gives me a gown with no back, tells me to remove everything and then get into the bed. After leaving most of my dignity on the chair next to Sandy, I lie back and wait.

A short while later, a nurse enters and starts my IV. Sandy does her best to keep me entertained but deep inside I am afraid. Having had nothing to eat or drink that morning, I am also hungry.

The transport staff enters to retrieve and wheel me down the hall to the heart catheter lab. They transfer me onto the procedure table and five or six personnel immediately surround me. One quickly slides off my gown while another begins rapidly shaving my groin. I am a bit too shaken by the experience to even care.

While lying there naked, my hip exposed, a technician walks by and jokingly says, "Hey look, we have a tattoo!"

Everyone turns and looks at my right butt cheek and the tattoo of my little dog's paw print. Up to now, this had been mostly a private matter. Now it is on display for all to see. In spite of everything happening, I start laughing.

They inject the sedative Versed into my IV. I remain somewhat conscious but care little about what is going on around me. They make the incision and insert the catheter which finds its way to my heart. I hear humming and clicking noises as well as distant voices, but I mostly drift along in a dreamlike state.

Toward the end of the procedure they inject a dye into my IV, one used for contrast. I was told earlier I would feel a warm sensation throughout my body after the injection. That is exactly what happens. In my drugged state, all I can think is "Wow – cool."

They finish the procedure and I am wheeled out into the hallway. I hear one nurse say, "I have never seen such clean veins and arteries in my life."

Even under the influence of drugs I wonder, Then why is this happening? I tell myself, the angiogram is supposed to provide answers.

I return to my room quite lucid, considering the usual amnesia-life effects of Versed. The nurse then tells me, "Don't move, lie flat and stay that way for the next two hours." The incision is sealed, but they want sufficient time to pass to ensure the wound is safely closed.

Sandy is waiting for me with a blueberry muffin to help quiet my growling stomach. I merely lie there and stare at the ceiling while she feeds the muffin to me. I notice she also brought with her a glass of water and a straw. I am so thirsty I ask for the water. I enthusiastically start to drink then realize that I cannot get out of bed to use the toilet. I also cannot sit up in bed and use a urinal. I immediately stop drinking the water and try to relax.

The two hours pass quickly with Sandy entertaining me. We talk mostly of our time spent in Needles and the funny moments we remember. The clock is ticking and my bladder begins to demand that I relieve myself sometime very soon. I close my eyes and try to think of anything but running water. I do not want a female nurse to come in, grab onto my manhood and point it into a plastic urinal.

The nurse finally comes in and tells me I can get up, dress and leave. I am still quite sore from the incision and move slowly. I dress and move as quickly as possible into the bathroom and to the toilet to relieve myself.

We leave the hospital to return to my home. I sleep for most of the afternoon since some of the drugs are still coursing through my system. I am proud of myself for successfully making it through what will be the first of many invasive tests and procedures.

Wednesday, November 4, 2009

I have always listened skeptically to opinions from the medical profession, large pharmaceutical companies and, especially, the government. Now, within a matter of a few days, I have been told my heart is dying and yet no one knows why. I know there is a reason and I also know I can find the appropriate treatment. No one is going to do it for me regardless of the number of degrees on their wall or the number of titles after their name.

My background is in engineering. Engineers view everything as a problem, and a solution exists for every problem. If you have problems with your approach it usually means you have problems with your design. Step back, reevaluate and start again.

So, I start reading. One book leads to the next. I am reading both sides of the heart argument but find the most compelling and complete information on the side of alternative or non-western contemporary treatment. There is a reason for heart disease, and there is an approach to wellness. I know I am heading down this path pretty much alone. And I figure I need to get a big stick because I face an uphill battle to get the treatment I need. If Dr. Michaels frustrates me this much already, what will I face when I start to make demands on different doctors? I am very frustrated and disillusioned with the medical machine. I don't think I am asking for all that much. I just want someone, at this point, to go over the possibilities and options. I want that "educated guess" I referred to earlier.

I have a large, wonderful, extended family, and I call my cousin Elizabeth who has an amazing background in nutrition and alternative approaches to healing. I know how she thinks, how she reasons and, because of this, I trust her judgment. She tells me to first read the book, "Iodine: Why You Need It, Why You Can't Live Without It" by Dr. David Brownstein. I go to his website and discover he has written many books and that he also writes a blog on current health issues. I order this book on iodine and read the summaries of his other books.

Because of my diagnosis, I find myself on short-term disability and have not only the time to read but also the motivation.

Thursday, November 5, 2009

I return to Dr. Michaels' office to hear the results of the angiogram. As before, he listens to my heart, my lungs, squeezes my ankles and says nothing more. He writes two prescriptions and stands to leave the room.

"Wait a minute," I say, "what about the angiogram? What does it show?"

He says with little interest or conviction, "Yes, you do have heart failure. Your heart is enlarged."

I already know that part, so I ask, "But why? Why is this happening?"

He answers, "We don't know."

I want to know why this man never volunteers information. Why is it my responsibility to squeeze data from him? Is this how he would like to be treated if in my position?

His final conclusion? My heart must have been attacked by a virus. There is no specific proof of this, it is just their best guess since they can't come up with anything more solid.

I'm frustrated and I go home knowing no more than when I first entered this man's office four weeks earlier.

Monday, November 9, 2009

I receive Dr. Brownstein's book and devour it in one day. I go back to his website and order two more books. Regrettably, I skip over his book, "Overcoming Thyroid Disorders." No one has mentioned anything to me about a thyroid problem. I do not know, as yet, of the strong connection between hypothyroidism and heart disease.

Tuesday, November 10, 2009

I go once more to Dr. Michaels' office for what seems to be the same, pointless routine. I learn nothing new and he offers no additional information. My meds are increased with little more explanation than what is offered on the bottle of pills I will later pick up at the pharmacy. Again, I feel brushed aside and ignored. I am also bored from being at home. I don't feel great, but I also don't feel overly sick. I ask Dr. Michaels for a release so I can return to work. He grants my request and I leave.

Monday, November 16, 2009

A week later, I return to work to continue my regular duties. I work in aerospace and test software used by the military. My job can be stressful but not particularly physically demanding. Even so, I am somewhat short of breath now and then; but all in all, I feel pretty good.

I try to ignore my problem and continue with my life as usual. As serious as my condition has been made to sound, I believe I can find the answers and find the best treatment. What I don't know, at this point, is how difficult it will be to find the right doctor.

Tuesday, November 17, 2009

While walking my dog in the afternoon, I run into my neighbor Mona. Mona's dog, Rocky, is a big, lovable chocolate Labrador and I am crazy about him. While playing with Rocky, I tell her about my heart issue and my search for answers and treatment.

She says, "Have you considered acupuncture?"

I hadn't but I am open to almost anything that doesn't include another synthetic drug. She recommends her chiropractor, Dr. Kris Kennedy, who also practices acupuncture. I plan to call him the next day.

Wednesday, November 18, 2009

I call Dr. Kennedy's office and am surprised when he personally answers his phone. I tell him I was referred by Mona and about my problem. I ask if he thinks acupuncture might help. He feels it is worth coming into the office and talking further, and I set an appointment for the next day.

Thursday, November 19, 2009

Dr. Kennedy is young, handsome, optimistic and enthusiastic. Quite a change from the dour demeanor of Dr. Michaels and attack attitude of Dr. Bailey. If nothing else, simply talking to him makes me feel better.

I give acupuncture a try. He leads me into a treatment room, has me strip and put on a gown. He reenters the room and begins covering my body with needles, my head, my face, my arms, my hands, and down to my legs and feet.

It isn't the insertion of the needles that bothers me; it is the idea of lying there with minimal movement for the next thirty to forty minutes that is unsettling. I take a deep breath, well, as deep as I can, all things considered, and try to relax.

Forty minutes later Dr. Kennedy returns and removes the needles. He sets me up on a schedule of treatments twice a week, dropping to once a week after the first month.

December 2009

Monday, December 7, 2009

After reading several books by Dr. Brownstein, I finally order his book, "Overcoming Thyroid Disorders" -- mostly out of curiosity. This book will mark the turning point in the focus of my treatment. Although I have been tested for hypothyroidism, Dr. Michaels hasn't indicated there is a problem.

In his book, Dr. Brownstein discusses hypothyroidism in detail. The thyroid gland is essential for the proper functioning of the body and the immune system. The link between hypothyroidism and heart disease is well known. Also, when the thyroid gland is not working properly it is not unusual for other hormone levels to also be low. In reading books by several doctors regarding hypothyroidism, I find that blood tests alone often do not reveal the extent of the problem. In addition to blood tests, patients must be evaluated based on physical symptoms. As I read through the list of symptoms, I can clearly see myself, my mother and my grandmother. (Please read "Overcoming Thyroid Disorders" by Dr. David Brownstein for a full list of symptoms and his recommended approach to overcoming this disorder. One other excellent book on hypothyroidism and its link to heart disease is "Hypothyroidism: Type 2" by Dr. Mark Starr.)

One important fact repeated in all of the books is that hypothyroidism must be treated with natural thyroid and not the synthetic form. The most common brand of natural thyroid is Armour. I now know what I need to take; now I need to find a doctor who will prescribe it. (Again, refer to either the Brownstein or the Starr books.)

I now have hope that something can be done about my heart failure.

Armed with this new information I am ready to talk again to Dr. Michaels to see what we can make happen together. I discover later that I am naively optimistic about his response.

Thursday, December 10, 2009

Three days later, I go to my regular appointment with Dr Michaels armed with several books and reports I have printed from the internet. I ask if I have been tested for hypothyroidism. Dr. Michaels assures me I have, so I ask to see the results of the test. Not surprisingly, I find my values are low but still in what is considered the "normal" range.

"Considering I have heart disease, wouldn't it make sense to raise these values to the high-normal range?" I ask.

"Why?" he replies. "The values are normal."

I tell him what I have been reading and why I am so interested in my thyroid tests. He looks at me blankly for a short while and replies, "If you want to see an endocrinologist, see an endocrinologist."

I am furious! So, let me get this straight, I think, you have no idea why this is happening to my heart, but what you do know, with absolute certainty, is that no other doctor, in spite of research with which you may not be familiar, knows more about heart disease and treatment options than you. In addition, you have no interest or curiosity as to what others may have found as successful approaches to treating heart disease.

I also want to ask him what percentage of his patients each year he actually cures, but I decide I probably know the answer to that question.

I know now I need to take even further control of my health and my treatment. No such support will be coming from this office.

Tuesday, December 15, 2009

About a week later, I run into Mona on my afternoon walk and tell her what I have been reading. She tells me she, too, suffers from hypothyroidism. When first diagnosed, her doctor prescribed the synthetic "non-FDA approved" thyroid medication called Synthroid. She took the drug but found little improvement in her health. Also, she had an allergic reaction to a preservative in Synthroid, and she felt aches all over her body as if she had been beaten with a bat. Mona was persistent and asked for a T3 and T4 test in addition to the T4/TSH tests usually run by doctors when searching for thyroid problems. The endocrinologist suggested Mona had fibromyalgia. Regardless of what her doctors were telling her, Mona did her own investigation and discovered her own path of treatment. She found the right doctor for her and recommended that I contact him. (Again, refer to "Overcoming Thyroid Disorders" by Brownstein for a complete explanation of the thyroid hormones, testing and treatment.)

Wednesday, December 16, 2009

I call the office of Mona's endocrinologist and ask to set an appointment.

"The doctor is not taking new patients," I am told.

Great. Now what do I do?

Thursday, December 17, 2009

The next day, while Dr. Kennedy inserts the acupuncture needles I tell him what I have learned so far about my condition and approach to treatment. He suggests another endocrinologist in the area who he feels might be willing to work with me.

When I return home, I call his office to set an appointment.

"Who is your primary care physician? Did he refer you?" I am asked.

"No," I reply, "I was referred by my acupuncturist."

She then says, "We do not make diagnoses here. You must have a referral from either your primary care physician or some other medical doctor."

My frustration comes out in waves. "Listen to me. I have heart failure and my cardiologist doesn't know why. My thyroid hormone levels are low. My basal body temperature is low which also indicates a thyroid problem. I need to see an endocrinologist and I need to see one as soon as possible."

She decides not to argue with me further and schedules me for the first available appointment. Unfortunately, it isn't until February 10th, almost two months from now.

Friday, December 25, 2009

It is Christmas morning and I can't think about anything other than my problem and finding treatment. I simply don't feel any holiday cheer.

My cousins Cindy and Sandy discover I have no plans and call that morning to invite me over for the afternoon. Part of me wants to sit home and be frustrated but I know I need to get away from everything for at least a day. I join the fun and feel a bit better.

Saturday, December 26, 2009

The day after Christmas, my roommate, Kevin, and I head to Palm Springs for a few days. The weather is perfect and it takes me away from home. I leave my books behind so there is nothing I can do but relax and enjoy myself.

Sunday, December 27, 2009

We get up early and take the tram to the top of Mt. San Jacinto. I had been there many years before and remember several easy walking trails around the rim of the mountain. What I don't consider is the altitude and the effect the thin air can have on my heart.

I exit the tram car, now at 8,500 feet, and my heart rebels. Every breath and every step are labored. We start walking through the chalet to the opposite side to where the trails begin. Any other time, I could easily walk down the path from the chalet to the trails. Today, I am afraid to even leave the chalet's terrace. I try to walk down a few steps, but stop at the first landing when I feel the tightness begin in my chest. I know this landing is as far as I will get today.

We reenter the chalet and make our way to the restaurant. We have lunch and return to the valley floor.

In the evening we leave the hotel for a two-block walk to a nearby restaurant for dinner. I think it is rather foolish for us to drive since it is so close. Still in denial of what my body tells me, we walk. I make it to the restaurant without incident but my return to the hotel is not as successful.

As we walk back to the hotel, I can barely breathe. It is the first time I begin to feel as if I am drowning. Finally, I stop and sit down in the middle of the block. Kevin offers to retrieve the car but my stubbornness doesn't allow it. It is only another block; it's no big deal.

I make it to the hotel realizing how sick I have become. I'm not getting better; I'm getting worse.

January 2010

Wednesday, January 13, 2010

Two weeks later my appointment with Dr. Michaels is the same as every other. No information, no change, no nothing.

Thursday, January 14, 2010

I continue working at my job but am feeling the negative effects of the disease. My commute is approximately forty-five minutes each way. I find it more and more difficult to function. By the time I get home in the evening I am so exhausted I can do little more than eat and sleep.

I can't last much longer.

February 2010

Monday, February 1, 2010

A month later, I decide I should probably take time off from work and just rest; maybe that's all I need. I look into temporary disability and make the necessary calls. I'm confident I will be back at work in March.

Tuesday, February 9, 2010

About one week later I receive a call from the endocrinologist's office. "Your doctor is not available tomorrow but another doctor in the group has an opening."

"I don't want another doctor," I say, "I want the one with whom I scheduled the appointment."

"Sorry, his next opening isn't until March," she tersely replies.

"Fine," I say with resignation, "I'll take the appointment tomorrow."

Based on my reading, most doctors are unjustifiably resistant to prescribe Armour Thyroid, so I am concerned about the outcome of tomorrow's appointment.

Wednesday, February 10, 2010

I meet with the backup endocrinologist and lay out my situation. I am armed with copies of my blood test results and several of my books.

He reviews the information and agrees to treat me. He writes me a prescription for Synthroid. "No," I say, "I only want Armour Thyroid."

As I expect, he is quite testy and refuses.

So I tell him to keep his prescription and I go home to start over.

Thursday, February 25, 2010

About two weeks later, in spite of doing little except hanging around the house, I am getting weaker and my symptoms continue to worsen.

Kevin, my roommate, and I discover we will have to move from our condo. The owners have let it slip into foreclosure and the bank is taking it over. We look for a smaller place which means I will need to sell much of my furniture. I also begin packing and throwing out stuff I no longer use.

Under normal circumstances, moving is stressful. For me, this seems to be an insurmountable task.

March 2010

Monday, March 8, 2010

I begin packing, fielding calls about the furniture I am selling, and I call trying to find a new place to live. I am tired and I feel terrible. But there is nothing I can do; these tasks have to be completed by the end of the month. Kevin works during the day and is unable to help.

We set the date of the move for Saturday, March 27. I begin calling friends for help, but most are busy. I can't imagine how I will be able to lift anything over two or three pounds. But I keep calling and finally assemble a small, but strong, group to help.

I keep getting weaker and now I am constantly coughing. My body is trying to purge my lungs of the fluid my heart is no longer able to move through and out of my system.

Wednesday, March 17, 2010

I see Dr. Michaels for my regular appointment and he gives me the news I don't want to hear. "We need to start considering a heart transplant."

This is a bad dream, I tell myself. I just need to wake up. This can't be happening to me. Tears roll down my cheeks. I am not the person who has heart disease, I think. They don't even know what is causing this. All I can do is quietly choke out, "Don't tell me that."

He tells me to contact the San Diego Cardiac Center. He says there are doctors there who can help me.

I leave his office numb and in shock.

Saturday, March 27, 2010

I try my best to wrap up what needs to be done before we move, before our friends arrive to help. My breathing is so labored I don't see how I can be of much help, but my ego won't let me sit and watch while everyone else works.

I try limiting my lifting to small, light objects. Moving up and down the staircase feels like struggling to hike in the thin mountain air. The pain in my chest continues to remind me how sick I truly am, yet I don't want anyone to know how badly I feel.

We load everything into the truck and head over to the new place. I am grateful for the twenty minute rest in the car, but I know I have nothing left inside to help unload the furniture and boxes.

I try to find things to do without actually lifting or going up the stairs, but those tasks are limited. I finally come across a light box that belongs in my new bedroom. This shouldn't be a problem, I think, I can handle this little thing.

By the time I get to the top of the stairs my lungs are on fire and I can barely breathe. I go into my new room and lie down on the floor, hoping no one will find me and panic.

My friend Steve sees me and rushes over, asking if I am alright. I don't want to upset anyone so I tell a lie and say I am a bit winded. I know Steve doesn't believe me; I'm sure he knows something is very wrong, but he just helps me up and tells me to sit, take it easy and not worry about moving anything else.

I am pretty much worthless the rest of the day. All I can think about is sleeping.

Sunday, March 28, 2010

I try unpacking boxes but my body, my heart and my lungs won't cooperate.

I also find it more and more difficult to lie flat while sleeping. It feels as if I am drowning and water is flowing into my lungs. I cough almost constantly as my body tries to rid itself of the fluid accumulating in my system. I try propping my head and chest up with pillows but can't find a position that works. I begin lying on the downstairs couch as it seems the only place where I can rest. I don't fall deeply sleep; I merely doze now and then.

I finally call the San Diego Cardiac Center and set an appointment in early June.

Monday, March 29, 2010

I wake at 5:00 a.m. hearing Kevin call my name. I am in my room, but kneeling at the side of my bed with my arms and head lying on the mattress. I don't remember moving into this position during the night.

"You've been coughing all night," he says, "I'm taking you to the hospital."

We drive to Mission Hospital. One thing I learn over the next few months is that when you enter even a crowded emergency room, saying the words "heart disease" gets you moved to the front of the line.

They take me to a room and begin running tests. They can clearly hear the congestion in my lungs and realize they need to act quickly. They inject Lasix, a common diuretic, into my IV and give me a urinal. In no time at all, my body begins releasing the fluids.

Within the next hour I lose over a liter of fluid from my system. The relief to my lungs is immediate. I am so desperate to feel better I don't even have the chance to be concerned about where I am or what this level of fluid retention might mean about the seriousness of my condition.

I am transferred to the cardiac unit and into a semi-private room. I need to sleep but my hospital roommate is agitated, angry and downright nasty to the staff. As sick as I feel and as badly as I want to sleep, his constant talking and complaining keep me awake.

I finally, quietly, ask my nurse if it is possible to move me somewhere, anywhere else. It takes a couple of hours but they find me a private room away from the angry man in the next bed and I am finally able to sleep.

Tuesday, March 30, 2010

Blood tests, x-rays and CT scans are the order of the day. But no new information comes to light. I have heart failure and my body is not functioning properly.

So, all they can do is treat the symptoms since no one knows the root cause.

Wednesday, March 31, 2010

I am released from the hospital and sent home. I feel pretty good, all things considered. I can breathe fairly well and I survived my first hospital stay.

Once home, I start unpacking and getting the house together. I am not sure how long this good feeling will last.

April 2010

Friday, April 9, 2010

I find myself doing little more than lying on the couch and watching television. My energy level is in freefall.

I now take Lasix every day to keep fluid from collecting in my body. I spite of this, I still have a mild sensation of drowning. I also find it takes little to make me cry. My emotions are out of control and it is something for which I don't much care.

Wednesday, April 14, 2010

About one week later, I wake at 4:30 a.m. in a panic. I sit halfway up in bed and pain quickly radiates through my chest. I let out a small yell. It feels as if someone is stabbing me with a dagger. I try sitting up further or at least lying back down, but any movement causes the pain to intensify.

Kevin hears me yell and comes into my room. "What's wrong? What's happening?" he asks.

"I don't know, but the pain in my chest is almost unbearable. I'm sure it isn't a heart attack, but I can't move."

"Should I call 911?"

Stupidly, I say, "No, help me out of bed, and I'll call Dr. Michaels' office in a short while and ask him what to do."

The pain finally eases a bit, and I am able to get out of bed. I shower, knowing I will likely end up back in the hospital. Whatever is happening can't be good.

Dr. Michaels returns my call and tells me to get to the emergency room immediately. He has already ordered a CT scan of my chest and they are waiting for me.

Kevin again drives me to the hospital. As we head up the street, he misses the first turn into the emergency entrance.

"Don't bother turning around," I tell him. "Just drop me off at the front of the hospital and I'll walk. Park the car and I will meet you inside."

The walk from the main entrance to the emergency room is farther than I realize. By the time I get there, the pain in my chest is so intense I am now walking bent over. As I enter the room I begin to collapse. A guard and a nurse rush over and I say, "I have a heart problem. Help me."

They rush me into the back and get me into a bed. Within moments I am hooked to various monitors and IV lines. A nurse asks if I want morphine. At first I say no, but later relent. But as she injects the narcotic, my blood pressure begins to drop. She becomes quite concerned and stops. She calls the doctor and I wait. Something is holding up the CT scan. I wait as the small amount of morphine I received takes effect and I feel some relief.

Suddenly the ER doctor and transport come into my room in a rush. I am quickly taken down the hall and into a lab for the scan. My body passes into and then out of the donut-shaped machine, and I begin to drift off.

As I am pulled out, the ER doctor is standing over me, ghostly white. He excitedly says, "Just lie there, don't move. Your lungs are filled with clots. It looks like someone took a paint brush and splattered red paint all across your chest. We are transferring you to a lab where they will go in through your groin and dissolve the clots. Just don't move. We are bringing in a pulmonary doctor, Dr. Goldberg, to handle your case."

It is amazing what you think and worry about in a crisis, how irrational you can be. I fully understand the severity of my situation yet my mind immediately runs to the irrelevant. When I first entered the emergency room I was given a gown and told to take off my shirt. They didn't ask me to remove the blue jeans I am wearing. Now being wheeled to the lab, I think, What about my jeans? These are new jeans, I like them. I don't want them cut off.

When I get into the lab they sit me up and slap defibrillator pads onto my back so should my heart stop they can shock it back into action. Four people come over and transfer me onto the procedure table.

I am still worried about my jeans. So, I ask the nurse, "Can I please take off my jeans?"

"No, lie still," she orders.

"But they're new," I beg, "I really don't want you to cut them off."

She finally relents and tells me I can undo the button and zipper and gently push them down around my thighs. Greatly relieved that, unlike me, my jeans will be spared the knife, I lose consciousness as drugs are injected into my IV.

They first insert an IVC filter which will catch clots, preventing them from reaching my heart and potentially killing me. The filter works as advertised and catches several before they are able to do their damage.

I stir from sleep as they wheel me into a room in the intensive care unit (ICU). I am transferred into a bed and my nurse comes over to settle me in. As she stands next to my bed, she rests her hands on my ankles. A look of surprise spreads across her face.

"Do you still have your pants on?" she quizzes.

"Yes, they were afraid to let me take them off earlier," I tell her.

"Do you want to keep them on?"

"No, please take them off."

The drugs from earlier still run through my system and I lie back and sleep. I have survived the first major crisis of my heart disease.

Death will have to wait.

Thursday, April 15, 2010

I am transferred from ICU to the cardiac telemetry floor and thankfully to a private room. The seriousness of the prior day's events starts to sink in. On one hand I am scared; yet on the other, I am trying to dissociate myself from what is actually happening. It is a defense mechanism, I know, but one that keeps me from totally falling apart.

I have a good stream of visitors, both friends and family, and they keep my spirits high. But I later learn just how sick I am looking and acting. My best friend from childhood, Robin, and his wife, Karen, come to visit. As a nurse, Karen cannot help but assess my situation, my speech, my skin color and my actions. They tell me much later that when they left my room, they did not get very far down the hall before they both began to cry. They knew I was dying.

Tuesday, April 20, 2010

The doctors discharge me. I am prescribed Coumadin, a blood thinner, along with the Lasix. The number of drugs I am taking is rapidly increasing. I am not happy about this but do not yet know of an alternative approach.

I am also fitted with a defibrillator vest. The vest monitors my heart and should the rhythm become erratic, the vest will zap me – hard. I hope it does not go off at some point for no valid reason; it would be quite the unpleasant experience.

Friday, April 23, 2010

It is almost impossible for me to sleep at night. I cannot lie flat on my bed so I spend more and more time on the couch, propped up with the television droning on. There always seems to be some sort of "Law & Order" marathon running through the night and I become addicted. Since I only sleep and wake, I find it difficult to follow the thread of the stories, but the stars of the shows: Jerry Orbach, Christopher Meloni and Mariska Hargitay, all become my best friends from midnight to 6:00 a.m.

My breathing is shallow and labored and, as the days drone on, it is more and more difficult to care for myself. I seem to be in a constant fog from lack of sleep and lack of energy.

My cousins Sandy and Cindy alternately stay with me. I remember sitting on the couch and talking to Cindy and in mid-sentence, I nod off. Minutes later I awaken and realize what has happened. This scenario plays out many times during their stay.

In the midst of this, Kevin finds a new job in Dallas, Texas. He begins packing and making preparations to move. I am concerned about being alone, but I also don't know who might move in with me.

I later discover I am not the only one worried.

Tuesday, April 27, 2010

The following week, I wake and sit up in bed. In the dark, I reach for the lamp and turn it on. I can't believe what I see. My forearms are huge, puffy and totally out of proportion to the rest of my body. Now what is happening?

I get up, go into Kevin's room and wake him. Seeing my arms, he, too, is alarmed. "We better get you back to the hospital. Something is seriously wrong here," Kevin says in a panic-filled voice.

Learning from my last crisis, I don't bother showering. We get in the car and drive to the hospital. At the emergency room desk I tell them I have heart failure and show them my arms. Nothing more needs to be said.

Knowing I have been treated for pulmonary embolisms, clots in my lungs, the doctors are quite concerned. They order an ultrasound of my arms and legs and find that both have multiple clots. The Coumadin is not working. My situation is getting worse.

What they do not know with any certainty is why these blood clots are forming.

After being in the emergency room most of the day, I am again admitted and transferred to ICU. I am tired, upset and discouraged.

Not knowing what else to do, Kevin tells the nurse I need to be bathed. Lying there in bed, I close my eyes and relax as the warm washcloths run over my skin. I want to sleep and I want to wake the next morning and discover this is all a bad dream.

Wednesday, April 28, 2010

My good friend, Jim, flies in from Florida to be with me. My aunt, Delores, comes down from the San Francisco Bay area and Uncle Bob and Aunt Peggy come from Rancho Cucamonga to sit with me. I probably have the best support group possible. Sandy also spends day after day sitting in my room. When they aren't chatting with me or amongst themselves, they are querying doctors as to my status and asking what more can be done.

Thursday, April 29, 2010

Kevin moves to Dallas, leaving me with an empty house in which to live when I return home, well, empty except for my little dog, Honey. In reality, I won't be returning home for quite some time.

The doctors put me on a more powerful blood thinner called Arixtra. The downside of this drug is that when I leave the hospital I must inject it myself into a fatty area of the body every day. Even though I have already dropped ten pounds, my stomach is still the logical choice. I will do this by pinching the fat of my stomach, stabbing the syringe into the area and pressing down on the plunger. The daily injection is something I really do not want to do and it is something I never do get used to doing. I just have to suck it up and do it anyway.

Even worse than the pain of the injections is what I learn next. Arixtra is expensive, very expensive. Even with my insurance, the cost to me runs about $400 a month.

Now I am feeling sick for multiple reasons.

Friday, April 30, 2010

My hospital groupies arrive early this morning. They want to be present when Dr. Michaels makes his rounds. When he arrives, they immediately begin pummeling him with questions. "Is he in the right hospital? Would a research hospital be better? Are there specialists who can be brought in?" They are relentless and I love it.

Sitting outside my room at his desk is the physical therapist who has been teaching me to walk with a cane. When all of my doctors finish their visits, he comes in to take me for my morning walk around the unit. "I couldn't help but overhear the questions your family was asking the doctors. Do you know how fortunate you are to have this kind of support system?" he asks.

"Yes, I do know," I reply. "I've always known. I have an amazing family and wonderful friends."

As days pass, walking becomes more and more of a problem. I feel as if in three short months I have gone from the age of fifty-one to somewhere late in my seventies. I look in the mirror and see the old man I am becoming. I am losing weight, I think partly from the steady diet of hospital food but also because I'm simply not hungry; I don't care much about eating.

Tests continue, one after another; now they are trying to find the reason for the clots.

At this point, I think I have been through just about everything until someone from transport comes in to take me for an MRI. Hmm, this should be interesting, I naively think. As they wheel me to the door, I smile and wave at my friends and family.

All of them smile and wave back, except for Jim. Jim has a rather concerned look on his face but says nothing. Jim is the only one in the group who knows what lies before me and he knows I have no reason to smile.

As I am wheeled into the lab, the technician asks me if I have problems with claustrophobia. I don't think so, but then, I have never been in an MRI before either. They give me a headset and ask what kind of music I want to hear during the procedure.

I throw them a curve ball. "I'd like to listen to Chopin piano music – the etudes," I say.

They look puzzled but go off in search of the music I hope will keep me calm.

I lie on the table which will slide into the MRI and am handed a "panic button" to use should I not be able to handle the confined space. I wasn't overly concerned about claustrophobia before, but now, holding the panic button, I am very concerned. I have seen this test on television; the machine isn't *that* small, is it?

All I can figure is people on television shows getting MRIs weigh only 35 pounds. The opening is so small that my arms have to roll slightly onto my chest and stomach for me to fit.

They locate M. Chopin and the music begins softly playing in my headset. The MRI is brought up to speed and the table moves into position. MRIs are loud, very loud, and the noise is unlike anything I've heard before. Also, unlike an x-ray or even a CT scan, an MRI takes time; in my case, almost forty minutes. The top of the inner tube is no more than one inch from the top of my nose. I close my eyes and try unsuccessfully to relax. Although the music is playing, it is continually interrupted by instructions to "inhale," "hold," and "breathe." I try to focus on the music, but with the constant interruptions, I begin to panic. I finally can take no more and repeatedly press the red button in my right hand. Get me out of here, I think.

They pull me out and I try to calm down. Clearly, I am not the first person to experience this. I take deep breaths and try thinking happy thoughts to slow the rate of my already damaged heart.

After a few minutes, I am ready to try again.

"Ok, forget the music, it doesn't help," I tell them.

I lie back down, close my eyes, and try to imagine myself lying on a beach in the Caribbean with the sun's rays warming my body, the sound of the waves lapping on the shore and the rustle of palm fronds in the breeze. It may sound corny or ridiculous, but with a lot of focus it works and I complete the test.

Upon returning to my room, I look at Jim with a now knowing look. He tells me later he didn't want to say anything. Anything he might have said would only frighten me. Well, I know one thing I will say to someone about to have an MRI, "Ask for drugs, lots of drugs!"

May 2010

After being in the hospital for about one week, the doctors are running out of tests to run and paths to take to find the reason for my heart failure and the associated blood clots. What to do? Everyone wonders. Treat symptoms, they decide.

By now, evenings are the worst. Anxiety attacks hit around 8:00 p.m. Even though my torso is propped up in the hospital bed, the sensation, probably from hypoxia: a reduction of oxygen to tissue, causes me to panic. I sit up in bed, turn and dangle my legs over the side and try to breathe slowly and deeply to calm down. This scenario plays out multiple times each night before I finally fall to sleep.

Thursday, May 6, 2010

It has been over a week and no doctor knows what more to do for me, so they send me home. But none of my family or friends wants me to live alone with my dog, Honey. Honey is my best little friend. I rescued her from a very bad area of Los Angeles after she had been badly abused by her prior owner. She is a mix of Chow Chow and probably Australian Shepherd. She looks a bit like a small golden retriever. She is very devoted to me, a one master dog. I am a little concerned about my ability to care for her living alone. Several friends and family members graciously offer me a room in their homes. I am overwhelmed by their kindness. My cousin Anna's offer seems the best. Their home sits on a large lot, roughly an acre in size. There are mature trees, flowers, shrubs, a fountain, and to top it all off, chickens running around in the back of the property. They refer to their estate as "The Ranch." In addition to the main house, there is a small bungalow in the back. It has a small living area, kitchen, bath and a bedroom. Since I can no longer sleep flat in a bed, a hospital bed is ordered. It is decided to place the bed, not in the bedroom, but in the front living area which is easily accessible. Also ordered for me are tanks of oxygen.

Anna comes this morning to pick me up at the hospital in her van. I'm sure it is a variety of things that trigger the attack, but I begin acting like I am crazy. Apparently, I am terrified of being discharged. The nurse says this isn't unusual, but her reassuring words do not calm me. I do not let Anna out of my sight. She wants to speak to the nurse outside my room but when she tells me she will be right back and starts to leave, I grab her arm and say, "No, please don't leave me!"

My mind knows I am acting like a lunatic, completely irrational, and yet I can't seem to stop myself. I am stressed and I am definitely stressing out Anna. Anna is also upset that the staff isn't providing help in how to care for me or telling us what to expect after leaving the hospital. Anna wants to know why they are discharging me while I am still so sick.

"What exactly am I supposed to do for him?" she asks the nurse.

"There is nothing more we can do for him here," the nurse replies.

I think we all wonder if I am being sent home to die.

In the midst of the panic and chaos I create, Anna makes the best executive decision possible. She looks at the nurse and says, "Get a wheelchair, we're leaving now."

I am put into the chair and quickly wheeled out of the room. Down the hall I go, into the elevator and before I know it, I am outside and being loaded into Anna's van. The amazing thing is, I go from totally panicked to totally calm. The attack simply stops. I sit back in my seat for the one-hour drive to Anna's house. I now have Anna, her husband Mike, and their four sons to watch over me.

I am so fortunate to have them there for me. On the other hand, I basically just want to go home.

Friday, May 7, 2010

It is the best possible arrangement. The bungalow is perfect. I have my own space, yet the main house is only steps away. I keep some food items in my little kitchen, but for the most part I eat with the family.

Anna is my cousin from my mother's side of the family, and we are all serious coffee drinkers. As I walk into the main house that morning, the rich smell of brewing coffee fills my senses. Yes, I think, smiling, this is going to work out just fine.

Anna comes out and pours us both a mug of the dark, rich, full-bodied, yet decaffeinated, brew. The boys are still asleep and Mike is busy getting ready for work. It is so calm and peaceful. It is the best medicine possible.

Monday, May 10, 2010

I begin settling into the routine in my little bungalow and in the main house. After living alone for so much of my life, it is rather fun being part of a family. The ages of the four boys range from seven to seventeen. Chris, son number two, and I get into the habit of playing gin rummy. I teach him how to play, and for a short time (very short) I am able to win regularly. But he catches on and quickly becomes good competition for me. At any time during the day he might look up at me, smile and say, "Gin?"

"Get the cards and prepare to lose," is my usual response.

Anna, like many in my extended family, is very focused on good nutrition. From their chickens they get organic, free-range eggs. She cooks an outstanding mix of foods that are all balanced, high in nutrition and low in sugar and bad carbohydrates. Yes, if I am going to get well, I think, this is the place where it can happen. Unfortunately, I am failing too quickly. Even life under the best of conditions, at this point, cannot make me better.

Anna's parents, my Aunt Peggy and Uncle Bob, live catty-corner from The Ranch. So I often take my cane and hobble over to their house for conversation and, what else, more coffee.

It is amazing how good I feel while, at the same time, feeling so bad.

Thursday, May 13, 2010

Anna drives me to Newport Beach this morning. Two weeks earlier I contacted the Whitaker Wellness Center for an appointment with Dr. Mark Filidei. I am hopeful he will be able to help me.

I look so old and frail and feel pretty much as I look when I meet with the doctor and he reviews my case. He prescribes Armour Thyroid and makes many suggestions regarding nutrients. He also suggests I take human growth hormone (HGH). Like the Arixtra I am already taking, HGH is very expensive and rarely covered by health insurance.

"Do you know how much this will cost me?" I ask.

"About $500 to $600 a month," he replies.

He also suggests treatments in a hyperbaric chamber.

I get the prescription for Armour Thyroid but tell him I will have to think about the rest. The costs, especially since I am now on disability, seem out of my reach.

During the hour drive back to The Ranch we talk about my next steps.

Friday, May 14, 2010

For over a month I have been experiencing something I cannot explain. Whenever I lie down to rest and am in that state between wakefulness and sleep, I sense the presence of a man. I cannot actually see him, but I begin talking aloud to him. I speak to him about 70% of the time in English and the rest in French. After many weeks I realize his name is St. John, pronounced in the British manner of "Sinjin." I do not remember the subject of my conversations with him, but Anna, Sandy and Cindy tell me I often laugh. When I do speak, it is sometimes coherent and sometimes not.

I later read a book about near-death experiences and how common it is for people to see and talk to friends and family who have passed before them. What is different about my situation is that I have no idea who St. John is. I do sense great comfort by his presence, though, and I guess no other reason or explanation is necessary.

Saturday, May 15, 2010

It is taco night at Uncle Bob and Aunt Peggy's house. The weather is perfect and they set up picnic tables in their back yard. My uncle browns and seasons the meat; and everything needed for the feast is laid out on the tables. The boys are thrilled, as everyone loves my uncle's build-your-own tacos. Well, everyone but me. I sit down, begin to eat and I think, these taste terrible. What's going on? How can everyone but me think they taste great? I politely finish my two tacos but remain puzzled as to why everything is tasteless. This isn't my family, I tell myself. Almost everyone is a good cook, and yet something is very wrong with dinner tonight.

Sunday, May 16, 2010

This next morning I discover it wasn't the tacos and it wasn't my uncle, it was me. My sense of taste is nearly gone. All I can still sense are very sweet and very sour foods. This is the first real sign of my system shutting down from the lack of blood flow.

I begin eating items, such as broccoli, which I usually avoid. It doesn't matter what I eat, nothing has flavor. I find I can only taste items that are very sweet or very sour. I go with Anna to the market and buy a jar of sauerkraut. I begin putting it on almost everything. Vinegar also becomes my friend at meals because it is something I can sprinkle on foods and sense the bite of the acid.

To satisfy the desire for sweet foods, I try frozen juice bars. Mike is good enough to go from store to store trying to find Welch's grape bars for me. He finds them and I keep them in the freezer in the bungalow. Every night before bed, I enjoy one grape juice bar. I chuckle about how my life has so radically changed. Before all this happened, an evening indulgence was a cigar and a good glass of scotch; now a popsicle puts the same smile on my face.

Tuesday, May 18, 2010

There is a new development in my continuing drama. My stomach begins shutting down. Suddenly my loss of taste seems irrelevant. Twenty minutes after eating, my meal comes back up. Anna is so wonderful, she tries preparing different foods for me, searching for something that I can keep down, yet nothing but chicken broth seems to work.

Wednesday, May 19, 2010

Every morning I weigh myself. Now that I am not eating, I expect to see a rapid drop in my weight, yet for some reason, it isn't happening. My weight remains the same.

Friday, May 21, 2010

My legs and ankles are now so full of fluid that the skin actually drapes down on my shoes. I begin wearing flip-flops because they are more comfortable and easier to put on and take off.

Sandy comes down and while looking at my swollen legs decides to take pictures and measure their size. My breathing becomes more and more labored and I am on oxygen 100% of the time. Even walking with the cane is difficult.

Friday nights are movie nights on The Ranch. Mike rents "The Black Stallion," one of my favorite movies. As the show begins, I realize I need to be in the hospital. I am so filled with fluid I can barely breathe. I begin feeling panic rising inside of me, yet I very much want to watch the movie!! Finally, I can take it no longer.

I turn to Anna and say, "I need to go to the hospital, right now."

Everyone jumps into action. My things are retrieved from the bungalow, I get into the car and they quickly drive me to San Antonio Hospital in Rancho Cucamonga. I am so weak and lightheaded, I can only get to the admissions window with help.

The emergency room is especially busy but I am rushed into the back. They start an IV and I wait. After considerable time, a doctor comes in and tells the nurse to start Lasix in my IV. But Lasix is now having minimal effect on me. I lose some of the fluid, but not as rapidly as before. Around 2:00 a.m. I am admitted to the hospital. I feel only moderately better and my legs look no different than when I was admitted. I seem to be losing the battle.

Saturday, May 22, 2010

I am not giving up fluid; the Lasix is not working. They try a more powerful diuretic and bring me a small pill. Within twenty minutes of taking it, it kicks in and I quickly begin to pee and pee and pee. I need more than one urinal next to my bed since I can easily fill up one and need a second before someone can come, measure and dispose of the contents of the first.

I am finally able to breathe again and begin feeling more like myself. I also discover why I haven't been losing weight the last weeks. What I have been losing in fat and muscle was being replaced by fluid. By the time I finally stop urinating, I have lost over ten pounds in less than twelve hours. Not a diet I will recommend to anyone.

I plead with the staff to release me. I do not want to stay in the hospital any longer than necessary. I want to go home, back to my bungalow. They finally give in and discharge me.

Monday, May 24, 2010

Several tests are scheduled for me for today to determine why I am unable to keep food down. Since January, I have lost about thirty pounds and am extremely thin. Plus, I am getting no nutrition in my body except for the broth Anna prepares for me.

The night before, I began drinking this white liquid and nothing else. Then, this morning, on the drive down to Mission Viejo I drink an additional bottle of the liquid. During the one-hour drive from Anna's to Mission Viejo, I unhappily sip and sip the unpleasant beverage until it is gone. What I really want is coffee. In spite of everything wrong with me, I can still taste and drink coffee. There is always a bright spot when you look hard enough!

The first test will be conducted in a lab in the same building as the gastroenterologist (GI) who wrote the order. It is a two-story, open-air building. We arrive early, and Anna and I sit outside to chat and stretch from the long drive. Having so much to drink on the way, I need a restroom. They are accessible from the outside court but I need a key. I walk into one of the offices, get the key, head to the restroom and relieve myself.

We still have about twenty more minutes to wait so we continue sitting and enjoying the morning air. Immediately before the test, I use the restroom one last time.

I unzip my pants and reach in for my penis.

I wish I now had a photograph of the look on my face at that moment. I am sure the look of shock and surprise was hysterical. I look down and see genitals that *must* belong to someone other than me. My penis is huge, and not in a good way. It is swollen and has an odd crick in the middle. Panic quickly sets in. I need answers and I need them fast.

I rush out of the restroom and Anna can tell by my face that something is very wrong. I am not quite prepared to discuss it with her and so I hurry into the office where the test is to be performed.

I tell the woman at the reception desk what has happened and ask if it is normal. She looks at me as if I am speaking a foreign language. She seems to just want me away from her desk. I'm sure the look on my face doesn't calm anyone near me either. She tells me to take a seat and says someone will be with me shortly.

A young man comes out and calls my name. He leads me to a small room and asks me to change into a gown. While changing, I again look down and see my swollen, deformed member. What is happening to me?

When I emerge from the test, I also ask the young man if this happens to most men. As with the woman at the front desk, he seems to want to do his job and get away from me.

The test completed, I change back into my clothes and walk out the front door. Anna is waiting and asks what is wrong.

"I've got to find a doctor and now!!" I tell her.

I walk across the medical complex to the office of my GI doctor.

I tell the young man at the front desk, "I don't have an appointment, but I just took a test ordered by this doctor. Something is very wrong with my penis and I need to see the doctor immediately."

Finally I have found someone who sympathizes with me. He quickly goes into the back, comes out and shows me into an examination room.

My doctor enters, I tell him what is happening and he says, "I'm not a urologist, I don't think I can help you."

"Look," I reply excitedly, "You ordered this test and someone's got to look at my penis and tell me what's going on!"

He reluctantly asks me to drop my pants. The look of surprise on his face is probably similar to the shock on my face in the restroom. He is momentarily speechless then says, "Has it always had that crick in it?"

"NO, it hasn't!! What's going on?" I beg.

"Hold on," he tells me, "I'm going to get you in with a urologist right now."

He leaves and returns with the address of a doctor whose office is close. I rush to that building and wait to be called. As I sit there I think, wouldn't it be ironic if by the time I see this doctor, everything is back to normal?

I am called into a room and as is typical, I have to explain my rather embarrassing situation to a nurse. The doctor enters and I again review the events of the last few hours. He asks me to drop my pants so he can have a look. He, reassuringly, does not have the same look of horror spread across his face as was on the GI doctor's. He tells me that because I was sitting in the car and drinking so much fluid, the liquid simply settled where I would rather have not had it settle. He says I am fine and the problem will clear up quickly. He does take one more look and asks, "Has your penis always had that crick in it?"

Relieved that amputation will not be necessary, we push on to another building and another test. The purpose of this second test is to determine how food is moving through my digestive system. In a small room, sitting on a table, is a sad looking sandwich made with white bread and scrambled eggs. I am told to eat the entire sandwich. I am not sure I will be able to keep the food down, as everything else I eat comes back up. Plus, the sandwich tastes terrible. I want to get the guy back into the room and teach him how to properly scramble eggs.

There is some sort of radioactive material in the eggs. This material allows them to perform a scan over the next forty minutes to see how it moves through my stomach and on into my intestines. After finally finishing the sandwich I am escorted to another room with a massive diagnostic device hanging over a table. I am instructed to lie down and the device is positioned over my lower torso. "Just lie still," I am told.

My mind races through all of the things that can go wrong. What if I have to vomit? What if I have to pee? What if I have another attack of claustrophobia? Happily, none of these things occurs. In fact, I am so tired from the events of the day, I actually nod off.

After spending most of the day in Mission Viejo, we finally drive back to The Ranch. Once back in my bungalow, my phone rings. It is my Aunt Delores in Northern California checking on my status. I begin telling her about my day, and as I tell her the ordeal about my penis I begin to laugh. Then she too begins to laugh.

"Isn't it funny," I tell her, "that men generally run around trying to protect and hide this part of their body, and here I was for several hours demanding someone look at it!"

My high spirits are short-lived.

Tuesday, May 25, 2010

The GI doctor gives me a prescription that once again allows me to eat without vomiting. Even though I can once again eat, I am still unable to taste food, which takes the joy out of my meals.

I continue growing weaker. My body is screaming at me to save myself, yet I don't know what more I can do. I am taking a tremendous number of prescription medications and nutrients each day, yet my health continues to decline.

Bedtime is a nightmare for all of us because that's when the anxiety attacks worsen. I often call Anna from the bungalow in a panic. She is always so sweet. She comes out and sits with me, since there is little else she can actually do. I lie down in bed, then bolt up, hang my legs over the side, pant, and often begin to cry. This can go on for fifteen minutes or as long as an hour before I finally sleep.

Although I am a very spiritual person, I am not a particularly religious person. But, with everything going on, I begin regularly praying for God to take me. I am not only ready to die, I want to die. I want to feel at peace again and it seems as if only death will allow it.

Wednesday, May 26, 2010 – Thursday, May 27, 2010

My pulmonary doctor, Dr. Goldberg from Mission Hospital, has scheduled me for a sleep study tonight to determine if I am suffering from sleep apnea which is often associated with heart disease. Uncle Bob and I first drive to my place in Aliso Viejo in the afternoon. While we wait, I doze off on the couch and he goes for a walk. As I lie there in my half asleep/half-awake state, St. John makes his final visit. While we are talking I am barely aware of how cold I am feeling. I begin to shiver but do not wake up enough to cover myself with a blanket. By the time Bob returns from his walk I am shaking badly. I lie in a tub of hot water to warm myself. This is the last bath I will take in a very long time.

After my bath, we go out for a late dinner. Around 9:00 p.m., Bob drops me off at the medical building where I will spend the night. He returns to my house to sleep, with plans to pick me up the next morning at 6:30 a.m.

I give credit to anyone in a sleep study who can actually sleep. Not only are you in a strange place, but you are hooked up to an unbelievable number of sensors attached to your head, face, chest and arms. You spend the night in a small, motel-style room complete with television, bed and items that attempt to make the room cozy. I am already quite tired when I arrive at the center and hope sleep will come easily. Considering everything happening in my life, it is a rather silly assumption.

Sleep does not come.

I try watching TV, resorting once again to Law & Order. I try lying in different positions in the bed but nothing seems to work.

At 2:00 a.m. I begin coughing. I am again filling with fluid and cough constantly. The nurse monitoring me comes into the room and asks what is happening. I tell her it is nothing unusual and not to worry. In spite of my dismissive attitude, she is concerned. She finally decides she cannot risk my health and calls the paramedics.

In no time the EMTs descend upon my room. There are eventually seven men and one woman crammed into that small area.

This is overkill, I think.

They start by taking my vitals and they notice my blood pressure falling. They, too, are concerned and make the decision to get me to the emergency room. They load me onto a gurney and take me downstairs to the waiting ambulance. I call Uncle Bob to let him know I am on my way back to the hospital and to meet me in the emergency room.

Amusingly, the hospital is only half a block away from the medical building. It is probably one of the shortest ambulance rides in history.

At 3:00 a.m., the emergency room is very quiet. They start the IV and take my blood pressure. It has dropped even further. They are also having problems sensing my pulse.

Uncle Bob arrives shortly. I need desperately to talk to someone, as I feel the end is near. Each time the automatic blood pressure cuff squeezes my upper arm the reading gets lower. The nurses and doctors are now extremely concerned. The numbers get so low that one nurse tells me she is surprised I am still conscious and able to speak. They then tip the bed so my head is lower than my heart in an attempt to stabilize the pressure.

I am alone with Uncle Bob in my room. He takes my hand to comfort me. I look up at him and say, "If it is my time, I am ready to go. I only wish God would act quickly."

I don't know how much time passes, but they finally stabilize me. I am taken upstairs to ICU once again. I am there one or two hours before Dr. Michaels enters my room. He reviews the events of the night, makes his assessment and says, "Tomorrow I am sending you by ambulance to Sharp Memorial Hospital in San Diego. I cannot risk your life any longer."

They then begin talking to me about the LVAD. Even though I am only half listening out of fear, I learn it is a mechanical pump that is connected to the left ventricle and the aorta. The pump brings blood from the ventricle around to the aorta and on to the rest of the body. Sharp Hospital in San Diego is known for both heart transplants and implanting LVADs. So, that will be my destination. As is usual, lately, I begin to cry.

The only explanation I still receive as to why this is happening to me is some mysterious, unexplained virus that must have attacked my heart. There is no proof, it is just the "best guess" available.

Friday, May 28, 2010

It is amazing how one remembers the smallest act of kindness. I wake this morning at 4:00 a.m. I lie there almost paralyzed by the fear of what is in store for me that day. My nurse sees my room light on and comes to check on me. I am his only patient that evening so he sits down to chat.

I tell him about the previous six months of my life and how they are now considering surgery to implant an LVAD. He listens quietly, aware of my emotions.

"Would you like a bath?" he asks. "Let me get everything together and wash you. It will make you feel at least a little better."

The bath is almost like a massage. He scrubs my entire body and even washes my hair. I feel better. I feel normal at least for a short while.

Through all my coming days and nights in hospitals, I will be extremely fortunate to have wonderful care by truly kind and thoughtful people. Yet for some reason, this nurse still stands out in my mind. It was exactly the right act of kindness at exactly the right moment.

Uncle Bob calls Anna and tells her I will be transported to Sharp Memorial Hospital. Anna drives down that morning to be with me. This is the Friday before Memorial Day and I know she and the rest of her family are leaving in the afternoon to drive to Cambria, about three hours north of her home.

Shortly after she arrives, a nurse comes to talk further about the LVAD. I know what lies ahead but I am not ready to hear the details. She has not gotten far into her presentation when I look at her and say, "Please leave the room, I can't hear about this yet. I don't want to know the details." My emotions are running at their peak. What I want to do is get out of the bed and run, but I have no energy left. So I lie there, while the nurse and Anna step out of the room.

While they are talking, the team from the ambulance arrives with their gurney. It is a driver, a nurse and one other young man to assist as necessary. Anna insists on driving down and meeting me at Sharp.

"Anna, no, please, I'll be alright. Don't make the sixty-mile drive to San Diego, you need to go home."

But Anna has already made up her mind; she is coming with me.

I am loaded into the back of the ambulance and we head out. All I can think of is the surgery and how quickly and radically my life has changed. The nurse and his assistant sit quietly in the back with me. I know I have to do something to distract myself or I will lose my mind.

"Would you guys please prop up this table so I can see you better?" I ask.

They kindly comply.

Once I am sitting up I say, "Look, I am frightened at what awaits me in San Diego and I need to talk. Not about the surgery or my health, I need you both to keep me distracted. Tell me about yourselves? Where are you from? How did you get into nursing?"

Both men seem a bit taken aback by my request. I'm sure most patients in an ambulance have no real desire to talk. But we have a great conversation, talking about travel, family, experiences and their future. The time passes quickly. But Sharp Hospital looms ahead and we soon arrive.

I am taken to the medical ICU floor and to my new temporary home.

My nurse, Pailai, comes in for her assessment. Pailai is absolutely beautiful and sweet, yet has a confident edge about her. Anna has not yet arrived and, although I did not want her to drive down, I also miss her and feel very alone.

Anna soon makes her way to my room. As I said earlier, it amazes me what I focus upon in the midst of a crisis. Anna had taken my clothes with her from Mission Hospital. We all know it is unlikely I will be leaving any time soon, so she leaves them in her car, knowing she will be back in the near future.

"Anna, I need my clothes and my belt," I tell her.

For all Anna has done for me over the last six weeks, I know she should politely refuse and say she will bring them another time. Instead, she makes the long trek back to her car in the parking structure and brings them to me. She then hugs me, says her goodbyes and leaves for the two-and-a-half-hour drive home followed by the three-hour drive to Cambria. And that assumes light traffic, something not likely on this particular Friday.

I feel a bit guilty but I also feel relieved that I have my clothes and, for some reason, especially my belt.

In a short while, Kristi comes into my room. Kristi is a nurse practitioner working with my soon-to-be new cardiologist, Dr. Peter Hoagland. Kristi also is beautiful, sweet and thoughtful. She and Pailai are both bright lights on a very dark day for me.

Kristi begins a very thorough assessment, asking multitudes of questions. As we talk, a phlebotomist comes in to draw blood. Since I am talking to Kristi, I am not paying much attention to what he is doing. But after a while it dawns on me that he has been there for quite some time.

I look down and ask him, "How many vials are you drawing?"

"I need twenty," he says.

At any other point in my life, this would shock me, yet that day it seems almost routine.

Kristi finishes her questions and leaves. Shortly thereafter another phlebotomist comes into my room to draws another fifteen vials of blood. I am tired and disoriented and too uncaring to protest. I do wonder if I will be rewarded with a Twinkie and a glass of juice, but quickly dismiss the thought.

Within thirty minutes, still another phlebotomist shows up to my room. Thankfully, Pailai is standing outside my door and stops her. "This man has been through enough today," she says firmly. "No more blood draws. You can delay these tests until morning."

Thank you, dear girl, thank you for looking out for me, I think.

Nature calls and I need to do something about it. I ring for Pailai and tell her I need to have a bowel movement. In ICU, the toilet is right in the room next to the bed. There is a curtain you draw around yourself but it still feels very awkward and a little too public for such a private event.

As I sit on the toilet I notice there is no toilet paper nearby. I look in a small cabinet next to me but find none. I call out for Pailai and tell her my dilemma.

"Let me go look for some," she says.

I wait and wait and wonder what is taking so long. I look again in the same cabinet and way in the back I find the last roll. Pailai finally comes back telling me she can't find any in the unit.

"No problem," I tell her, "I did find a roll."

After getting back into bed I ask her how it is possible that there is no toilet paper.

She smiles and says, "You have to realize that right now you are the only patient in this unit who can use the toilet on his own."

Saturday, May 29, 2010

Today is the parade of the "ologists." Every thirty minutes or so, a different doctor enters my room. It starts with the cardiologist, followed by a hematologist, then an endocrinologist, an oncologist, and so forth. With this many doctors assigned to my case, I now understand why so many blood tests were ordered the prior day.

Just when things begin quieting down, Dr. Robert Adamson enters my room. Dr. Adamson is the surgeon who will perform my operation to implant the LVAD. My sister-in-law is an operating room nurse and over the years has told stories of surgeons that made me concerned about who would be operating on me, and what did I know or not know about him. I know nothing about Dr. Adamson, but when he comes in and introduces himself I look up and think, Thank you, God, for sending this man to care for me.

I have immediate confidence in him and I know I will be alright.

My cousin Sandy makes the seventy-mile drive from her home to Sharp Hospital to be with me this morning and to try her hand at beating me at gin rummy. As we play cards the nurse comes in and tells me I am being transferred to the cardiac floor. My things are gathered and I am wheeled to an elevator and on to my new room. Sandy spends the better part of the day with me making a difficult situation much easier. Since Sandy is a nurse it also makes me feel safe as she watches every movement and action of every hospital employee entering my room. As sweet as Sandy is, I feel a little sorry for anyone who might make a mistake around her. I know she would not hesitate to point out the error and ensure it is corrected. Two months later, in a different hospital, I will witness just how demanding she can actually be.

Sandy finally needs to head home and leaves me. For whatever reason, during all of my stays in the hospital, I do not want to watch television or even read. I don't know why neither appeals to me. So I lie quietly or sometimes doze off.

I do have some small glimmer of hope that somehow, someone will have an answer or approach that does not involve surgery. But I also know I am dying and I am running out of time. I know it is unlikely anyone will find an alternate solution, but still I pray for a miracle.

It is impossible to explain to someone just how badly you feel when you have heart failure. Every system in your body is operating at reduced capacity because of reduced blood flow. So you feel bad all over, yet can't always explain why. Plus, the sensation of drowning never fully goes away. You cough and cough and cough but nothing changes. As much as I fear the surgery, I also look forward to feeling normal again.

Monday, May 31, 2010

Tests continue to be ordered, each demanding more blood, more scans and more x-rays. Once again I am taken for an angiogram. I feel I can do nothing more than simply submit. I have little fight left in me.

Kevin flies in from Dallas to spend time with me. He is able to work remotely, and fortunately Sharp has WiFi throughout the hospital. There is a couch in my room and he sets up base and keeps in touch with his office.

The hospital maintains an office of nurses who work only with LVAD patients. It is around this time I meet Suzanne and Marcia: two important members of my team who help me through this ordeal. Both are rays of sunshine that I need right then as the reality of the surgery looms ahead.

I suspect I will be operated on later this week, although no one has actually said as much. Part of me simply wants it over, and anxiety keeps building in my stomach.

Tomorrow will be June. In my life, it will be, to paraphrase FDR, a month that will live in infamy.

June 2010

Wednesday, June 2, 2010

Surgery is set for Wednesday, June 9, a week from today. What are they going to do with me for a week? I wonder. In spite of being so weak, I do not want to spend the next seven days simply lying in bed.

When the doctor comes in to visit, I ask if I can go home over the weekend. On Saturday, my grand-niece will have her first birthday party and my entire family will be present. I can't help but worry that I might die during surgery and I want to see everyone before that day. This is the perfect opportunity.

The staff is reluctant to let me go, yet give in. I can leave tomorrow, but I need to be back early Monday morning so preparations for surgery can begin.

Thursday, June 3, 2010

I am free! Kevin drives me to Aliso Viejo. The place is still in a minor state of chaos since neither of us has been present to put things away; but it doesn't matter, I am home.

Saturday, June 5, 2010

Kevin drives me to my brother's house in Yucaipa for the birthday party. Yucaipa is about one and a half hours from Aliso Viejo. My brother and sister-in-law have hosted many of our family gatherings. I am grateful to have been born into a family with lots of aunts, uncles, cousins, nephews and nieces.

Natalie, my grand-niece, was born three months premature under difficult circumstances. Not only is she a tough little fighter, she is also adorable and sweet and loves to laugh. My brother has three large dogs and they run around greeting everyone and keeping Natalie amused.

I hobble up the walk from my car. At this point, I am already horribly skinny, having lost over forty pounds. I am walking with a cane, I drag an oxygen tank with me, I wear a defibrillator vest, my skin is a grayish color, and, in general, I look like death. No matter, the little girl makes me smile and we sit together in the rocking chair and rock. It is the best gift I can possibly receive.

It is difficult returning home that afternoon. Not only did I leave those I loved, I am also afraid I might not see them again in this life. June ninth is now only four days away and I am scared.

Sunday, June 6, 2010

Kevin's flight to Dallas is in the evening, but I need to be back at Sharp early tomorrow morning. Kevin calls friends who live near the hospital and makes arrangements for me to stay the night at their house. Tomorrow, they will drive me to Sharp.

I pack the few things I need, including my computer and my cell phone, and away we go. We arrive at Rey and Maricris' home in the mid-afternoon and sit and visit for a while. They have two young daughters, twins, who run around and entertain us. No matter how badly I feel, dogs and children make me smile.

We go out for dinner and by the time we get home I am quite exhausted. I go to my room to lie down. It is difficult for me to sleep under the most ideal circumstances, but here I am in an unfamiliar place on the night before I am to reenter the hospital for major surgery. I fortunately asked Rey how to tap into their WiFi and I spend most of the night on my computer, both on the internet and playing card games. I try to remain distracted, keeping my thoughts away from the next few days.

Monday, June 7, 2010

The night is long but morning still comes. I shower, for what will be one of my last times, have breakfast with the family, gather my things and Maricris drives me to the hospital.

She drops me off at the front entrance, gives me hug which I desperately need and drives away. I reluctantly and slowly walk into the hospital to the admissions office. I am numb as my senses continue to shut down, unable to fully deal with the events ahead.

Admission goes smoothly and I am escorted up to my old home on the fifth floor. I change into the gown, set my personal items aside and get into bed.

The usual routine begins of starting the IV, taking my vitals, listening to my heart and lungs, and documenting everything.

My nurse today is Laura. She is a tiny bit of a thing somewhere around my age. She is a joy to be around yet is very no-nonsense. She is the right nurse for me at exactly the right time.

There have been so many things about the next few days that I fear. I have needed to talk to someone about the details, but for some reason have not yet felt comfortable enough with anyone to actually ask. It is as if God has sent Laura to me this specific day for just this conversation. I know some of my concerns are silly in the grand scheme of things, but maybe I again focus on the trivial to avoid thinking of the seriousness of the actual events. The enormity of the surgery and what my life will be like afterward is too much to digest. Laura sits with me as if I am her only patient, her only responsibility that day, and she helps me through some of my fears.

Laura also helps me with another nagging problem. For all the discomfort I have endured during different tests, what really bugs me is the daily EKG. Each morning a tech comes in, hooks up leads to my chest, runs the test, then one by one, rips the leads off. Now I'm not a furry bear but I'm not smooth either. The pain of having the hair ripped from my chest each morning is getting to be too much. Also, the IV has to be moved every three or four days and that involves ripping tape off my arms and with it the hair that resides there.

"Laura, could you get a shaver and get all of the hair off my chest and arms?" I ask.

She does, and I feel much better. It is a small change, a small event but at least I know for the next week or two the morning EKGs will be far less painful.

Laura is an angel. I will never forget her kindness.

Tuesday June 8, 2010

I begin to understand the difference between fear and terror. I have known fear and now I know terror. What I am now experiencing causes my senses to dull and in some cases, even shut down. Preparations start for my surgery the following morning and I submit to each request as if in a daze. I have no desire to know why things are happening, I simply accept and comply. My nurse today is Lisa, another special gem. I feel concern and compassion from Lisa as if I am her brother or uncle.

I am so weak and I find each action so difficult that I rely more and more on the staff for help. I feel ashamed that I can do so little. Lisa comes in with disinfectant towels for me to wipe over my body. She leaves the room so I can have privacy, but I find I am unable to complete the task alone. Simply leaning down to my legs is more than I can accomplish. I call her back and ask for her help.

I still feel I may not survive surgery. I have no real regrets in my life; there is no business I feel needs to be completed, yet I also feel compelled to make three phone calls, one to each of my nephews. I need to let them know how much they mean to me, how much they have meant to their grandmother, and how much I want them to have full and joyous lives.

The fog of the day does not lift. Sandy, Jim and Mary all come to stay with me. I know they are there yet I remember nothing else. At the end of Lisa's shift, Lori, also a wonderful, caring nurse, comes on duty for the night. Lori tries as best she can to make me comfortable. I am so tired, tired from weeks of not enough sleep. I begin to nod off, yet the moment my head falls back I wake with a start and sit up. I am again hit with attacks of anxiety and, like so many times before, I sit up, dangle my legs over the side of the bed and try to calm myself. The first storm passes and I try again lying back, trying to relax. Jim will tell me later he prayed for me, prayed I would sleep. But sleep is elusive that night.

Jim and Mary finally say their goodbyes, but Sandy stays with me through the night and on through the next day. I finally fall asleep, but well after midnight and it will be only a few short hours before I will be awakened.

Wednesday, June 9, 2010

I vaguely recall some of the final preparations before surgery. As I am wheeled out of my room, Pailai, my nurse from ICU, is there wishing me well. She has heard this is the morning of my surgery and comes to the cardiac unit to see me. I am touched by her thoughtfulness.

I am taken to a holding area before entering the operating room. Sandy is still by my side and takes several pictures of me. In the photos, my eyes are open, yet I am so drugged and dazed I later remember none of it.

Sandy stays at the hospital while I am in surgery. The surgeon periodically comes out and gives her status of the operation. Sandy then calls Anna who sends e-mails to my friends and family.

I later read those e-mails and will be struck by one in particular. After the device is implanted, the surgeon waits about thirty to forty minutes before closing my chest to let the pump run to ensure everything works properly. I can't help but wonder what the surgical team does during that time. Step outside for a cigarette? Run down to Starbuck's in the lobby? Do they cover my chest with wax paper, Saran Wrap, or a damp towel?

Everything is working as advertised and my chest is closed. They inform Sandy I am doing well and she goes home after a very long two days.

Thursday, June 10, 2010

Tonight I meet who I will later refer to as Handsome Mike. Why that becomes his nickname, I'm not quite sure. Mike is handsome, but Mike is also quite a character. Mike is a nursing assistant and although not assigned to me, comes in and sits and talks with me in the middle of the night. Mike is thinking about going back to school to get his RN. I push and push as much as I can.

"Yes, that is exactly what you need to do and the sooner the better," I tell him. "You will regret it if you don't go."

I pray for Mike and for his successes. My night nurse is Marcus, again the right nurse for me at the right time. Marcus is young and strong and makes me feel safe. I am so weak and frail and having this guy who looks like he could lift me right out of bed in one motion makes me feel better. Each night for the next several days, I lie in bed and hope Marcus will be my nurse again that evening.

Slowly, through a thick fog I am aware I am alive and aware my cousins Anna and Ruth are in the room. I am still intubated and I am aware I cannot talk. I first try gesturing, to indicate I want water. When they don't understand my hand motions, I switch to signing, using the alphabet of American Sign Language. Sadly, no one in the room but me knows the signs. Anna and Ruth try to guess the letters and I point at them when they guess correctly. But in a short time, I am once again unconscious.

Later that day the breathing tube is removed. My throat is quite sore and my mouth unbelievably dry. But, I cannot be given water. Anna and Ruth take turns standing next to my bed. They apply chapstick to my lips and are able to take a small sponge soaked in water and rub it across my teeth and lips. My mouth is so dry I quickly close my lips on the sponge, trying to suck out just a few drops of the precious liquid in a weak attempt to slake my thirst.

I try to speak but fall back asleep midsentence.

Anna and Ruth leave at the end of the day and spend the night with friends in San Diego.

I remember only brief moments of what is happening. I do recall in the evening, about every three hours, two nurses come over to my bed, grab hold of the sheet and pull me higher onto the mattress. Over time, my body slides down and this puts me back into the proper position. Next, one nurse leans across and tips me slightly to one side while the other slips pillows under my back. I tense up, afraid of the pain when they pull on my torso. Shortly thereafter, I quickly slide back into night.

Friday, June 11, 2010

When Ruth and Anna come to visit this morning I am more alert, but I have amnesia-like symptoms. I talk to them, although not always coherently.

I keep thanking them profusely and also, after asking for one thing or another I say, "I'm sorry."

Ruth finally tells me not to say, "I'm sorry" any longer.

I, of course, reply, "I'm sorry."

The television is turned to a music channel and pictures of flowers and mountains and streams display on the screen. I comment to them how beautiful everything is. They both tell me later that I was quite funny that day.

I also keep asking when my brother will arrive as well as one of my nephews.

Late in the night the hospital staff get me up and out of bed. It takes three guys to keep me up and hold me in place so that I don't tip over.

Saturday, June 12, 2010

I wake as if dreaming. Someone is lightly touching my hand. I slowly open my eyes and see my brother and my three nephews standing next to me. It is the first real moment of clarity since surgery. Seeing them, I smile, partly because I realize I am okay, that I have made it through the worst of the ordeal.

Both this day and the next are days I will never forget. Friends from all over southern California come to see me, often driving hours to get to Sharp. I am overwhelmed by their love.

At times I need to sleep but I don't want anyone to leave. My dear friend Jennifer makes the two-hour drive from Long Beach bringing with her an adorable stuffed black bear to keep me company.

My body finally gives out and I ask everyone to leave. I have so many reasons to be grateful, so many reasons to smile. And finally, after so many weeks of sleeplessness, I sleep.

Sunday, June 13, 2010

I am actually feeling great. I cannot believe how quickly I am mending considering it has only been four days since the surgery. The parade of friends and family continues. I'm sure there is probably a visitor limit in surgical ICU but no one enforces it. I am very animated and talkative and I guess they see no need to clear the room.

I start to realize one very interesting thing about myself. I am not a total introvert but I am definitely not what you would consider to be an extrovert. I'm not afraid to talk to people yet I rarely initiate conversations. But I have been a different person during my stays in the various hospitals. I am very outgoing and friendly to the staff, often complimenting nurses and technicians on their smile or personalities. I have endearing nicknames for many of them. I refer to several of my nurses as "my angel." I believe it is my way of coping with my own fear. If I make things seem light and happy then maybe they actually are, maybe none of the bad stuff is happening. Or it could be common sense, being nice to people wielding needles and knives.

As I lie there, I begin to take stock of all that has been done during the operation. I can see the base unit of the LVAD with the tether line running underneath my top sheet. The tether connects to the controller unit lying next to me on the bed. From the controller, a line runs under my gown and into my side where it then connects to the pump attached to my heart. There are also three drains coming out from just below my heart, each running to a separate container lying beside my bed. Of course, I still have an IV line into which various medications and fluids are fed. I also have a catheter which I try to ignore.

Sunday is a big event; I am finally allowed to drink water. But no one simply hands me a glass and a pitcher and tells me to have at it. One of the side effects of having the breathing tube down my throat for so long is the irritation it has caused. This then affects my ability to swallow. There is concern I might choke while drinking liquids. So, the solution is to add a thickening agent to all liquids. Lumpy, gooey water, mmmm… what a treat that is! But it gets even better. Soon I am also drinking lumpy, gooey chicken broth. They aren't ready to bring food, which actually doesn't bother me. I don't even want to think how solid food will be served. I can only imagine something like Gerber baby pureed carrots or something of the kind. For now, lumpy water is fine.

Monday, June 14, 2010

Kristi comes to check on me. Her smile and personality are infectious. She smiles so I smile. She tells me that everyone is thrilled with my progress and they will likely remove the first of the drainage tubes later that day. Looking back, I should have knocked on wood or done some other superstition-type action because her prediction doesn't quite work out as planned.

Later in the afternoon, a friend from Orange County comes for a visit. Shortly after he enters my room and begins to chat, an occupational therapist comes in and wants to talk to me. She sits down and asks if I might need help relearning various daily activities such as brushing my teeth, bathing and so forth. As we chat I notice her eyes drifting to the center of my chest.

At first I think nothing of it but then she says, "Is that blood on your gown?"

I look down and see a small spot consisting of blood and bodily fluid. "I think one of the drains might be leaking. Could you please call the nurse and see what she wants to do?" I ask.

Before she can even rise from her chair, the blood and fluid begins to push outside the drain and down my stomach and gown. Then the pain hits. I begin to writhe in my bed as staff rushes in to deal with the problem. I try not to scream but the pressure is terrible and I begin to moan. The pain briefly eases and I hope the worst is over. But it isn't and the scenario replays itself.

My friend stays, trying to comfort me, but he becomes emotional about seeing me in so much pain and I have to ask him to leave. I can't handle my problem as well as him being upset. I need to be alone with the nursing staff.

My nurse, Enjoli, a sweet, beautiful young woman, is there with me through the entire ordeal. Even after her shift ends, she stays. She remains with me until everything is under control and I am comfortable. She is definitely one of my many angels.

I lose over a liter of blood and fluid during the crisis and it is necessary to give me a blood transfusion. They are finally able to control the problem but the ultimate solution is worse than the actual event. They tell me another drainage tube will need to be inserted into my side tomorrow to further reduce the fluid buildup which caused the pressure and the leak.

My intuition tells me to be concerned. My intuition also downplays what lies ahead.

Tuesday, June 15, 2010

The morning routine in ICU is most annoying. At 3:00 a.m. a technician rolls in his portable x-ray machine and gets a shot of my chest. One hour later, just as I start to fall back asleep, the lab tech comes in for blood draws. This is followed by the regular check of my vitals and an EKG. Periodically they throw in an echocardiogram for good measure.

After this morning's routine is complete, the transport team enters to take me to a CT lab. A doctor and his team are waiting. They will insert the new drainage tube into the right side of my lower torso. I am transferred to the table and lie on my left side. I face waist level to several technicians assisting in the procedure. I am given some sort of drug, but am still awake. The doctor begins the insertion and the pain immediately radiates through my body. It is horrible. I try to speak but I can barely get out a whisper.

"It hurts," I say. But because of the noise of the machines, no one can hear me. I finally will myself to move my right arm up near my face. The technician standing there has his arm resting on the table in front of me. I am finally able to grab hold of him. He quickly looks down at me and I repeat, "It hurts."

"I know it does," he replies, "but we can't give you any more meds. You'll just have to take it."

If there is a bright side to all of this, it is that the procedure doesn't last long. I return to my room, grateful it is over and hopeful nothing more will go wrong.

Enjoli is my nurse again today. Late in the afternoon she comes in and says, "We can remove the catheter now."

I look at her and say, "No."

Puzzled, she looks at me and is unsure of what to say.

"I can't let you do that. You are too sweet and too beautiful. Your removing the catheter will make me feel like a dirty old man. Is it possible for a male nurse to take care of this? It is nothing against you, it is my problem, but please humor me."

She is wonderful about it. She calls in Steve, a male nurse who took great care of me the two days after surgery, and the catheter is quickly removed.

I guess because I interrupted the normal flow that day, no one mentions the need for me to drink a lot of water. The reason becomes apparent at the shift change.

My night nurse arrives at 7:00 p.m. She is the one nurse who cares for me at Sharp with whom I don't seem to click. She is a bit distant, not unfriendly, but not friendly either.

She checks my chart and says, "Have you urinated since the catheter was removed?"

"No, not yet. Why?" I ask.

"Because you need to pee within the next sixty minutes or we will need to reinsert the catheter," she replies.

Re-insert the catheter? While I'm awake? Oh no, no, no. I grab the water pitcher and begin to drink. But there isn't enough time for it to flow through me. As the clock ticks away, I try everything I can to squeeze out a drop or two. Finally, with fifteen minutes to spare, I am able to start the flow and I put some liquid in the urinal.

I call the nurse and proudly display my accomplishment.

She looks at the urinal and says, "It's not enough. You'll need to do better."

Looking at the clock and knowing the current state of my bladder, I know it isn't possible. I gave her all I could for at least another hour or so. She leaves my room and never says anything more about reinsertion.

I sleep with one eye open, thinking she might return and do the unthinkable. She doesn't; I am fine.

Wednesday, June 16, 2010

Each day I feel better and better. I can't believe how much better I feel and look since having the LVAD implanted. My grey skin is pink again, I can taste food, my stomach is processing food and on and on.

There is talk of transferring me out of ICU and on to the cardiac floor, but the final decision is made to wait until Thursday.

Suzanne visits me today to review the LVAD equipment and check on my progress.

"Is it possible for my heart to heal and reach a point where I will no longer need the device?" I ask.

"It is possible," she replies, "but at present, only one percent of Sharp patients have reached that point. Usually the pump is in place until a heart transplant is performed. Or in other cases, the LVAD is in place for the rest of the patient's life."

I decide I like the "one percent option" best. That is my goal. I feel I am on the right track from my reading and my contact with Dr. Filidei. When I leave Sharp and return home, I will return my focus on what is necessary to repair my heart. I will find my path and one day I will return to have the device removed.

One interesting note about LVAD patients, we don't have a pulse or a blood pressure readable by the standard procedure. Instead, a Doppler device is used along with the pressure cuff. It is very odd to reach down to your wrist and no longer feel a pulse. I can't help but wonder if I have entered the realm of the walking dead.

I am eating again but I have to pay close attention when I swallow, especially solid foods. It isn't unusual for the food to get into the back of my throat and then stop. It takes two or three attempts at swallowing to actually get the food down.

My physical therapist comes to get me up and walking. This is quite a task considering the number of tubes and receptacles attached to my body. He brings in a walker and begins the process of hooking each item to its sides. This is the first time I try my hand at disconnecting the LVAD from the base power source to batteries. It is a rather simple A to A and B to B connection, but I screw up on my first attempt. Thankfully, everyone is patient and forgiving. I don't walk far and it takes more effort than I realize. I have spent so much time in bed and have been so inactive that my muscles are weak. I shuffle out to the nurses' station, turn around and come back to my room and my bed.

Late in the afternoon my nurse and a nurse practitioner come to see me. The NP announces she will be taking out the first of the drains. For whatever illogical reason, that frightens me. She asks if I want some morphine which I gladly accept. My perception is that this process will be quite painful.

As she prepares to remove the drain I look up at my nurse and say, "Will you please do me a favor? Will you hold my hand?"

She is so sweet and seems a bit touched by my plea. She gladly holds my hand and I once again discover I have been very worried over nothing. The drain slips out easily with no pain or discomfort. I once again survive a crisis that exists only in my mind.

Thursday, June 17, 2010

I am finally moved back to the cardiac floor and all of my nursing friends. I settle back into the "old" routine, one that no longer includes a 3:00 a.m. x-ray. Blood draws still happen at 5:00 a.m., but I am often awake by then anyway.

My parade of visitors slows and I miss their company. Yet now and then someone surprises me and drops in. My good friend and hair stylist, Jay, comes down and even cuts my hair in the room. I have gotten pretty shaggy during my stay and am glad to have my hair short again.

The nurses are wonderful about washing my hair, but it is quite an ordeal and I always feel hesitant to ask.

Each day I feel a little better and gradually each drain is removed. Even after knowing the process is basically painless, I am still a little squirrelly each time it happens.

I have met my new cardiologist, Dr. Hoagland, on two or three previous occasions. His personality is somewhat reserved but I feel I am in good hands and am always happy when he comes by. But this day, I am especially happy to see him.

Because I am still on a diuretic, I take potassium each morning. But the protocol states that should the level of potassium in my blood get too low, I am to be given more through my IV. No one warns me of the effects of potassium given through an IV or even when they are adding it to the bag. As the potassium finds its way from the bag, down the tube and into my arm, a searing pain strikes. I immediately call for the nurse and ask her to do something.

Today, it happens again and as before, I am not sure why.

When Dr. Hoagland enters my room, he finds me ringing for the nurse and growling, trying to cope with the discomfort. He comes quickly to my bed, trying to determine what is wrong.

The nurse enters shortly and Dr. Hoagland asks, "What have you given him?"

"Potassium was added to his IV," she replies.

"Can't you see this man is in pain? Why are you doing this?" the doctor demands.

"Because it is in the protocol," she says.

It is Dr. Hoagland's reply that forever bonds me to him. "Well the protocol is stupid!"

I am no longer given potassium in my IV. It is administered orally. Each day, life gets a little bit better.

Sunday, June 20, 2010

As I continue to improve, I want more and more desperately to return home. My room has a great view and from the window I can see the freeway below. It seems what I want most is to drive again; I guess in some way being able to drive means freedom to me.

Each day the physical therapist takes me for longer and longer walks. The final test is for me to walk up and down a flight of stairs. My body is ready but my mind wants to hold me back. I am afraid of the most basic movements. But finally I am triumphant in my descent and ascent of the stairs, and thus ends my hospital physical therapy.

I have two more wickets to pass through.

First I am to leave my room and have lunch in the cafeteria. Second, I am to leave the hospital, with a friend driving, for one additional meal. I cannot be discharged until I have done both.

Monday, June 21, 2010

I am now feeling well enough to also be bored and antsy. I have had quite enough of hospital food, being stuck in my bed for most of the day, and am ready to get back to a normal life. This frustration makes me somewhat sullen.

It appears I will be discharged on Wednesday. Getting everything in place to go home is quite a logistical task. The Ranch is two and a half hours north of Sharp so Anna will need to make arrangements to come down early to take me home. Being discharged from any hospital is always an ordeal and it never seems to happen as planned. Mission Hospital has an amusing sign in each room stating the importance of "checking out" by 1:00 p.m. The only control a patient might have in meeting that deadline is if they permanently "check out." If 10:00 a.m. is the target for your discharge, plan on 3:00 p.m. to actually leave.

Uncle Bob and Anna come down on Tuesday to take me to my required lunch in the cafeteria. Then on Wednesday, we will leave the hospital to have the dinner. I should be discharged later that evening and I will be on my way home.

Ah, the best laid plans......

Tuesday, June 22, 2010

Everything is moving forward perfectly. My family comes down and we all head to the cafeteria for lunch. I dress in real clothes for the first time in weeks, get my walker, and begin the long, very long, as I discover, trek to the dining hall.

As we enter the cafeteria, my senses are hit with the smell of barbecued spare ribs. After weeks of hospital food, I think nothing can possibly smell better. Yes, I will have ribs and baked beans and salad. I am almost giddy.

It is a perfectly beautiful June day in San Diego and the cafeteria has an outdoor terrace. We all settle at a table and start lunch. The ribs are actually quite good. In fact, they are so good I want to go back for more. I revel in the feeling of being normal again, but the feeling is short lived.

Suddenly, my hearing drops by about half. Everything sounds dull and muted. Then I begin feeling lightheaded. I know I am about to pass out. I tell Anna how I feel and put my head between my knees. Anna calls to the nursing station in the cardiac unit and they rush down to meet me.

By the time they reach me with a wheelchair, I feel a bit better but also very tired. I am glad to get back into my bed and I want to sleep. But before I can nod off I can't help but wonder if this will delay my release. Being discharged is at the very top of my priority list.

Around 4:00 p.m., a nurse comes in to give me a onceover. Shortly after surgery, I started wearing boxers under my gown. I didn't want to be concerned with accidentally flashing other patients or staff. As she looks me over she notices a small amount of blood on my shorts which could only have come from my rectum.

When she mentions it to me I say, "It's nothing, please don't tell anyone. I'm okay." This will only interfere with my release and pointless begging seems appropriate.

But, it is her job and duty to report her findings which then set in motion events I would rather avoid. An endoscopy and a colonoscopy are ordered. This means I will need to drink that nasty liquid for the next several hours completely cleaning out my system. The experience is unpleasant and slightly degrading. When I have no more waste to give, I am taken to a lab, they knock me out and one tube is inserted down my throat and the other tube also finds its intended target. They discover nothing, but the process delays my release by one day.

Wednesday, June 23, 2010

I am not a happy camper. I am supposed to go home and instead I am being held captive. I am still required to go out for dinner before I can be released. Our plan was to do both the lunch and the dinner on the same day. But, obviously, that didn't happen.

Anna, Uncle Bob, Aunt Peggy, Anna's son Chris and I, all head to Chipotle for dinner. I merely want to get through the meal; I don't even enjoy myself. I want tomorrow to come quickly and to go back to my little bungalow on The Ranch.

Thursday, June 24, 2010

This is the big day. I am finally being discharged. As I stated before, the process takes time, lots of time. I don't realize how much stuff I have accumulated at the hospital until we start to move everything. In addition to things I brought from home, I now have the equipment needed to keep the LVAD running properly. They bring in a cart to my room and we begin to load it up.

As happy as I am to leave, I have formed bonds with those who have cared for me. I am a little sad. These people have meant so much to me and now I am leaving and I know it is unlikely I will see them again. But it is time to return to my life.

Anna goes down to bring her car to the hospital entrance. It takes one person pushing my wheelchair and another following with all of my belongings. Everything is loaded into the van and I then get out of the wheelchair, sit down in the passenger seat, and buckle up.

The door closes and Anna turns to me and says, "Where do you want to go?"

Without a moment of hesitation I reply, "In-N-Out Burger!"

I think she knew I was going to say that as she smiles and drives away from the hospital.

Oh mercy, that burger is so good, and along with it I have a strawberry milk shake. But what is most important is that I am going home.

The two-and-a-half hour ride passes slowly. The Ranch seems so far away. I can't help but think of all the times my family made this long drive to the hospital to be with me and how fortunate I am to have them as part of my life.

We finally pull into the driveway of the house. Mike and all of the boys come out to help. Everything in the car needs to be removed and hauled back to the bungalow. The LVAD equipment also needs to be set up and readied for me.

I have also bonded with the bungalow; it is a safe place for me. I walk slowly to the back of the property and to my little home. Anna and Mike's youngest son, Sam, made a sign that hangs on the door: "Welcome Home Tom!" On it is a drawing of my little dog, Honey, with whom I will be reunited the next day.

I sit on the couch, look around and begin to cry once more. The nightmare is ending, although not completely over. As I sit there, everyone begins to filter in: my aunt, uncle, the boys, Mike, and Anna. The room isn't designed to handle this many people so I suggest we all move back to the main house. It is getting close to dinner time and Anna has work to do.

It has been a long day. After dinner I realize just how tired I am.

I stand up, thank everyone and say, "I'll see you in the morning, I need to get some sleep."

Anna tells me later it was a very odd moment for her. I simply went alone to the bungalow and went to bed. No more anxiety attacks and no more phone calls asking her to sit with me. Much of the drama of my first four weeks at her house is now over.

Well, it is only over briefly.

Around 1:00 a.m. Friday morning, another mini-crisis hits. One thing I didn't consider is that I am still on a diuretic and am no longer in the hospital. I wake with a panicked feeling of needing to urinate *immediately*. But unlike at the hospital, there is no urinal sitting next to my bed and I am tethered to the LVAD base unit. Although the cords are long, I have not tested to see if they are long enough to reach the toilet.

I get out of bed, grab the lines and start to walk toward the bathroom. They don't reach. I feel like a three-year-old child needing to pee so badly he begins to dance. What do I do? I look around for something to use as a urinal but nothing is close enough. What is close is the front door of the bungalow. If it comes to that, I can step outside and water the plants. Ok, that calms me slightly; I have a viable Plan B. I try one last time to see if I can get the tethers to reach the bathroom. I find if I run them under the door and I stand at an angle, I can just barely hit the toilet with my stream. There is nothing quite like that feeling of relief.

Tomorrow, I will figure out how to properly deal with this situation before the next night. For now, I go back to bed.

Friday, June 25, 2010

Never has there been a morning so sweet. I get up, disconnect from the base unit and onto the batteries, walk over to the main house and as I walk in, the aroma of freshly brewing coffee fills my nose. Ahhh….. home. For the month I spent in the hospital I had nothing but what I consider a "coffee facsimile." But all that is forgotten as I pour my first cup of heavenly Joe.

Saturday, June 26, 2010

My focus is now on life with the LVAD and the changes this requires. Rule number one: don't get wet. So showering and bathing are both out. When I left Sharp, Anna thankfully grabbed three of the small plastic basins that were in my room and brought them home. I now fill two with warm water, add liquid soap to one, and take a sponge or bed bath. Not very satisfying, but it is my best and safest option for staying clean.

There is actually a way to shower with the device. Suzanne, my LVAD nurse, reviewed the process with me one day in the hospital. But she also warned me that water is the biggest reason for infection. Water from the tap may be safe to drink but it isn't sterile. There is currently a gaping hole in my side where the drive-line, the power source for the LVAD, exits my body. My skin has not yet closed around it. My fear of a systemic infection, which would land me back in the hospital, is my deciding factor in not even attempting to shower. I just got out of the hospital; I have no intention of going back in any time soon.

In Anna's laundry room is a large, deep washtub. I find I can bend over the sink and easily wash my hair. The entire process of washing myself and my hair takes time, but it also makes me feel normal, something I haven't felt in quite some time. It is also nice taking some sort of bath without an audience, unlike in the hospital.

I think I feel great, but my body is weaker than I want to admit. I sleep eight to nine hours a night but still need a two-hour nap in the afternoon. I do walk around the property now and then, but it isn't enough.

Because my chest was completely opened during surgery, I am not allowed to drive a car for another four weeks. It is also not wise for me to walk my dog, Honey. She tends to pull on her leash and that, in turn, pulls on my chest. So, Anna's son, Chris, assumes dog-walking duty for me.

I didn't care for the bag the hospital gave me in which to carry the controller and the batteries. It seemed a bit too small and awkward. So, while I was still in the hospital, I found a messenger-type bag on the internet and ordered it. It is leather, wide enough to hold the controller and the batteries and also all the paperwork I need to carry with me at all times. It is waiting for me when I arrive home. I transfer the equipment to the new bag and use the other as the backup. Wherever I need to go, this small bag containing two spare batteries and a spare controller goes as well. I begin calling it "the football" after the satchel of nuclear codes which follows the president of the U.S. That soon becomes the name by which everyone refers to it.

Tuesday, June 29, 2010

I settle in to a routine and am feeling better each day. I am now anxious to go out with friends and have dinner. Kevin will be coming for a visit over the weekend and I set up an evening for Kevin, two friends of ours and me at a restaurant near downtown Los Angeles. It will be a pretty big outing, but I feel I am up for it. Plans are set for Friday, July second.

July 2010

Thursday, July 1, 2010

Kevin arrives at The Ranch in the afternoon after his flight from Dallas. Since I am not using the bedroom in the bungalow, he moves in.

We all gather in the main house and have dinner. It is wonderful. It seems that all of the bad is behind me and everything going forward will work out well.

Back in the bungalow that evening, Kevin begins asking me questions about my stay in the hospital. To the surprise of both of us, I begin crying, no, more like sobbing. I know Kevin must wonder what exactly he said to trigger this, but it wasn't him. It is as if all the things in the hospital I simply "toughed out" and all of the fear I suppressed, now comes out. It feels good to release it all.

Friday, July 2, 2010

In the late afternoon we get ready and leave for our dinner in LA. It is a pretty big deal for me, my first real "field trip" in several months. I think I am ready, I feel good and I am excited to go.

We meet our friends at the restaurant at 6:00 p.m. The menu is filled with wonderful French delicacies and I have trouble deciding which to choose. I am flying high, life is good again. But it suddenly becomes too much for me. I realize halfway into the meal that I am running on limited energy. Shortly after I finish my main course, I apologize and excuse myself. I tell everyone I have to lie down and probably sleep. I take the car keys from Kevin and go out to the car to rest.

Kevin is so thoughtful. Everyone orders dessert so Kevin makes a plate of a little of each one and brings it to me in the car. Everything is wonderful, but I know I need to get home and into bed. I am completely spent and now know with certainty I am getting ahead of myself. I need more time to heal and to do what is necessary to make my body stronger.

Thursday, July 8, 2010

I plan to return home to Aliso Viejo in about two weeks so I also begin thinking forward to what will be necessary to make that happen. I will be alone and I try to determine if that poses any problems. I will probably be more comfortable if someone is there with me, but I can't think of anyone who might fill that role.

Well, God is looking out for me and the most amazing thing happens. My friend, Susan, a coworker from years before, has wanted to move from Palm Springs down to my area, and wants the chance to look around before settling in one place. We talk and she happily agrees to move in with me for a few months until I am stronger and more sure of my health situation. It is a great relief having that load lifted. We decide she will move in shortly before I return home. Kevin's furniture is in place in his room, so she only has to bring her personal belongings.

I am very thankful and relieved.

Monday, July 12, 2010

After breakfast I walk over to Uncle Bob and Aunt Peggy's house and join them for their morning coffee. While we chat I suddenly feel odd, the same feeling I experienced in the cafeteria at the hospital. My hearing shuts down and I know I am about to pass out. I drop my head between my legs and wait. Slowly my hearing becomes normal and the lightheadedness passes. The episode is over, yet I still do not feel quite right. I excuse myself and walk back to the bungalow to lie down.

Tuesday, July 13, 2010

I can't understand it; I'm not gaining any weight. Anna is feeding me like a farmhand and yet I am still skinny as a rail. I weigh myself every morning and at six-foot-six my weight hovers around 180 pounds, still fifty pounds below my weight of only five months earlier. I avoid looking at myself in a mirror because I am so horribly thin.

Another change: apparently from the trauma and the drugs of the prior month, my hair has started falling out. Every morning I resist washing or combing it because of the loss. I can't help but wonder if baldness is a very unwelcome side effect of the medications I am taking.

Wednesday, July 14, 2010

I still want to get out and see people but cannot yet drive. One thing I begin to discover is that once you've come close to dying, but survive, everyone wants to take you out for either lunch or dinner. It is wonderful side bonus.

I have not seen my good friends Richard and Natasha in a long time. We decide they will come to The Ranch on Friday and they, my cousin, Cindy, and I will go to a local restaurant for dinner. It sounds perfect.

Thursday, July 15, 2010

I feel a little odd today, as if I am coming down with a cold. I pretty much stay in the bungalow and do nothing. After my nap in the afternoon, I feel pretty good again. Whatever was wrong seems to be gone.

Friday, July 16, 2010

Richard, Natasha and Cindy all come over and we sit and chat with Anna and Mike before heading out to dinner. I feel strange again, but can't pinpoint exactly what is wrong.

We drive the short distance to the restaurant, are seated and begin looking at the menu. I begin feeling cold even though it is summer and the restaurant is not running its air conditioner. Richard drove us to the restaurant and I ask him if he has a jacket in his car. He does and retrieves it for me. We order our meals and shortly thereafter I begin feeling nauseous. I go into the restroom but nothing happens.

I return to the table and reluctantly begin eating my meal. I am feeling worse every moment and in spite of the jacket, still feel cold. I finally tell everyone I need to lie down. I take Richard's car keys and curl up in the back seat. They hurriedly finish their dinners and drive me home. By now I am shivering. I call down to Sharp Hospital and they tell me to get to an urgent care office for evaluation. Anna wants to take me directly to Sharp but I am not sure I can handle the trip.

Anna calls my cousin, Sandy, and fills her in on my situation. Sandy also wants me to go to Sharp. Because of the instructions I received over the phone when I called Sharp, I tell Anna to take me to a local urgent care first, to see what they say.

By the time we get to the urgent care, I am shivering like a Chihuahua in the snow.

I am taken to an examination room but when the doctor sees me he says, "Get him out of here; he belongs in a hospital."

One limitation of the LVAD is I can only go to hospitals with LVAD programs. That limits my options in Southern California to Cedars Sinai in Los Angeles, Sharp in San Diego, and Loma Linda Hospital. Since Loma Linda is the closest, we go there.

Although they have an LVAD program, they have done only one such surgery. I am quite the novelty in the ER. Doctors keep stopping by my room asking to listen to my heart. Of course, what they hear isn't my heart so much as the hum of the pump connected to it.

I finally vomit and continue being extremely cold. The reason is quickly discovered. My temperature is now over 104 degrees. No matter how many blankets are over me, I am still cold. I am admitted and taken to a room while Anna drives home to pick up my LVAD equipment.

So, I am back in the hospital. Loma Linda is fine, but it isn't Sharp. I am sorry now that I didn't listen to Anna and Sandy and head to San Diego immediately. But, there is nothing I can do about that now. It is almost midnight; they start me on antibiotics and I fall quickly to sleep.

Saturday, July 17, 2010

My fever continues. They determine I have a strep infection but considering I haven't had a sore throat earlier, they don't know how it got into my body. They test the area of the drive line but it comes back negative.

A nurse comes in with two bags of ice and tells me to hold them under my arms. It is the oddest sensation having them there but they do little to lower my body temperature. As they continue to monitor me, my temperature rises close to 105. So far the antibiotics are not working and I am getting weaker.

The decision is made to bring in what is called a cold blanket. It is a plastic drape within which water flows. It is connected to a base unit that cools the water and pumps it through the blanket. They bring it in and place it on top of me. Oh, one more thing, to keep me from getting too cold, my body temperature has to be constantly monitored. This is accomplished with an unpleasantly placed probe. I finally feel some relief and in spite of all that is happening, I am actually able to rest.

Monday, July 19, 2010

It is finally determined from the cultures which course of antibiotics to give me. Sandy is there with me, again keeping a close eye on my care. A phlebotomist enters my room to draw blood, not fully knowing who is witnessing her every move. Sandy asks her which tests are being run. She tells Sandy the names of the tests and draws two vials.

She leaves my room and Sandy says, "Those should be two separate draws from two different locations. She didn't do that."

Sandy goes out into the hall, retrieves the phlebotomist and has her redo the blood draw. Sandy also calls down to the lab to report the error.

I'm not making friends at Loma Linda but I am also too sick to care. At one point I scheme as to what I can do to get myself transferred to Sharp. I feel safer there and I would be cared for by people I already know. But, it is not to be.

Tuesday, July 20, 2010

The proper antibiotic is discovered and added to my IV line. I begin to feel the results quickly and again want to get out of the hospital and back to my little bungalow. But no one is yet ready to release me.

Thursday, July 22, 2010

Two days later, the doctors reluctantly agree to send me home. They initially want to insert a line in my chest by which I can continue injecting the antibiotic for several more days. I protest and beg them to let me continue on oral medications. They finally relent and discharge me.

Another minor nightmare is behind me.

Wednesday, July 28, 2010

I am finally going home, home to Aliso Viejo. Susan has moved into my place two days earlier on Monday and is waiting for me. Sandy comes to Anna's in the morning and we load her car. I am stunned at all of the stuff I have amassed. Her trunk and back seat are completely filled.

I am ready to go home, yet I also am sad to leave. Anna and family have taken such good care of me and I know I will miss the meals together, playing cards with the boys, talking, laughing and walking next door to have coffee with my aunt and uncle.

Sandy drives me home and she and Susan unload everything while I sit and watch. I am pretty much weak and worthless. After they finish, I notice it is time for lunch. I have been craving so many different foods for so long and right now I want Chinese. There is a great place not too far from my house and I offer to treat them. Sandy quickly says she will drive.

"Nope, not today," I say. "I'm driving." I have waited so long to get behind the wheel of a car and I am not going to be denied.

We have a wonderful lunch and I feel fantastic.

Thursday, July 29, 2010

I am now adapting my routine from being at Anna's to being back in my own home and that includes preparing my own meals. Although I like to cook, it was rather nice not having to make any food decisions while at Anna's. Now, the ball is back in my court.

I also need to figure out what I need to eat to gain weight. During my stay in Loma Linda I lost another three pounds.

So, I go to the store, and in addition to my usual items I pick up ice cream and other high calorie foods. Even if they aren't especially good for me, they still might add pounds to my frame.

August 2010

Wednesday, August 4, 2010

I've had the LVAD for about two months now. What is my day like living with it?

At night I sleep with the controller unit--a small white, plastic, oval box with two buttons and six lights--next to me in bed. The speed of the pump is set through the controller but can only be set at the hospital by the LVAD staff. Usually the speed is between 9200 and 9800 revolutions per minute (rpm). There is a line that runs from the controller into the side of my body up to the pump which is connected to my heart. The other end of the controller has two lines. These are connected at night to a base unit which is plugged into a wall socket. In addition to the base unit there is a battery charger which can charge up to four batteries at once.

Upon waking, I disconnect the controller from the base unit and plug into two of the batteries. These are kept at the side of my bed in a bag that I carry with me during the day. I put the seven-pound bag around my neck and shoulder, leave my bedroom and go into the bathroom. After first using the toilet I prepare to bathe. I use the two plastic basins I took with me from the hospital. I fill both with warm water and add an antibacterial soap to one of them. Using multiple washcloths, I scrub myself first with a soapy one and follow with one rinsed in clean water. Around my waist is a band, which I'll describe shortly, which has to be loosened and held in place while I wash around my torso, avoiding the dressing under which is the drive-line. Once bathed, I towel dry.

Next is my hair. When I first got home, I began washing my hair in the kitchen sink. This worked well, but was inconvenient. I later found a way, using a removable shower head, to wash my hair and lower body in the shower without getting my torso wet. I then dry my hair, brush my teeth, shave and so forth.

Twice a week, today being one of those days, I change the dressing around the drive-line. To do this, I surround myself with everything I will need and lie back in bed. First I don a surgical-type mask and latex-type gloves. Around my waist is a band about four inches wide, held closed with Velcro. On one end, the center is split open. This opening lies above the actual drive-line site and dressing. On top of the band, the drive-line is slightly coiled in the manner of a shepherd's crook and held securely by two Velcro straps attached to the outside of the band. This is done so that should the attached controller drop, there is some resistance and protection for the actual entry point of the drive-line.

Once the band is removed, I then remove the outer, circular dressing. Beneath that dressing is a small rectangle of material made from silver. This further protects the site from infection. I first open a packet containing what looks like a large safety match or a small popsicle. The end is a soft material saturated with an antiseptic solution. I clean my skin around the entry point with each side of the wand. After letting my skin dry I take a new rectangle of silver and apply it around the line. The next packet is a no-stick solution on a much smaller wand. This is applied around the silver to provide a barrier between my skin and the adhesive of the outer dressing. Once applied, a new circular dressing is placed and secured around the line. A new band then goes around my stomach; it is then closed and the drive-line secured to the outer layer.

I now dress and am ready for the day. I sit on my bed to relieve pressure from the strap around my shoulder, remove the strap and put on my shirt. I then put the strap back into place, stand and put on my pants. The drive-line from the controller runs discreetly from the bag, under my shirt and into my right side. But, one last check of my batteries. I press one of the buttons on the controller and one to four lights illuminate telling me the amount of power left in the attached batteries. Should the battery power get too low, an alarm will sound, warning me I have fifteen minutes of battery power remaining. When this happens I immediately replace the current batteries with ones fully charged. Based on the power level in the morning, I can roughly gauge at what time during the day the batteries will need to be changed. But, I can never leave the house without taking with me "the football," the bag containing two spare, fully-charged batteries and a spare controller.

With something around your neck weighing seven pounds you don't easily forget its presence. It may suddenly shift forward as you lean to pick something up or the strap may begin falling off your shoulder. Dropping the controller is the worst possible scenario. The sudden tug can cause the drive-line to rip open the entry site. This warrants an immediate call to the LVAD team at Sharp. This is also the most common reason for infection in LVAD patients. An infection will generally land you back in the hospital.

In July 2010, Vice President Dick Cheney also had surgery to implant the Thoratec Heartmate II. Often when I am changing my dressing I wonder, Does Mr. Cheney do this himself, or is he fortunate enough to have someone do it for him? Like me, he lost a lot of weight during his ordeal but in recent television interviews, he looks his usual self again. I wish him the best in his life with the device.

As each day passes, the process fades from an annoyance to merely routine. I have, although, never really gotten used to changing the dressing. There is just something a little creepy about seeing that line coming out of the side of my body.

Tuesday, August 10, 2010

Today I return to the Whitaker Wellness Center for my first appointment with Dr. Filidei since my surgery.

Now that I am feeling somewhat normal and out of danger, I need to address the core reason behind my heart disease. Dr. Filidei proposes high doses of several nutrients along with Armour Thyroid, daily injections of human growth hormone and semi-weekly injections of testosterone. Since self-injecting the blood thinner Arixtra, I am reasonably comfortable with the process. It is also around this time I am taken off Arixtra and switched back to Coumadin. Since I no longer have that $400 monthly expense of Arixtra I feel I can handle the cost of the human growth hormone treatments.

I set up two weekly pill boxes to organize my medications and nutrients. This way I do not need to measure each dose daily and I can easily take the pill boxes with me when I have a meal away from home.

I continue to read books on heart disease and other health issues and begin making changes to my diet. The more I learn about foods and how they affect health, the less I want to eat in restaurants and especially fast food joints. This means I am preparing more and more of my own meals.

Although I do enjoy cooking, meal preparation seems never-ending. I start thinking about ways I can cook and freeze balanced meals. I discover I can buy ten or twelve different vegetables and chop them finely in a food processor. Then for two or three days I make soup, spaghetti sauce, meatloaf, and several other dishes. Each dish contains a generous portion of the vegetable mixture. Everything is then frozen in individual meal-sized packets for reheating later. I can make somewhere between thirty-five to forty meals in one session All meals are high in animal protein, high in animal fats and low in all carbohydrates except for those from vegetables. I always reheat the meals in a pan on the stove, never in a microwave oven. Microwave ovens change the vitamin content and availability in foods along with the structure of the amino acids. Blood profiles of people regularly eating microwaved foods are similar to profiles of people with early stage cancer.

This works out well for me. Not that I eat this way exclusively, but the meals are quick and easy and far more nutritious and balanced than any store-bought frozen dinner.

Friday, August 20, 2010

Although Dr. Hoagland is now my primary cardiologist, I still have appointments with Dr. Michaels: my original cardiologist in Mission Viejo. In general, I meet with Dr. Hoagland every three months and with Dr. Michaels during the two months in between. This is to limit my driving to San Diego to only four times a year.

Dr. Michaels' routine never changes. He listens to my lungs, to my heart and then pinches my ankles. He says almost nothing to me and, for the $40 co-pay, I begin to wonder why I bother with the visits.

Sunday, August 22, 2010

My friend Gary calls and invites me to lunch. It is one of the many free meals my ordeal has earned me. I have not seen Gary since May, but more importantly, he has not seen me. On my way to the restaurant to meet him, I realize I have not warned him about my appearance. I weigh only 177 pounds. In spite of my hearty diet, I am still not gaining weight.

When I enter the restaurant I see Gary sitting at a table with his back to me. I walk over, touch him on his shoulder and greet him. He stands and turns to say hello. The look on his face says it all. Gary is rarely at a loss for words but now he is silent. My face must have looked like it belonged to a ghost or the walking dead. I tell him it is alright, that I am ok. Yes, I do know what I look like and the best thing for me to do right then is to eat! We have Korean barbecue that day and stuff ourselves with lots of red meat and pickled vegetables. It is wonderful and I hope it will be good for at least an additional pound or two.

Monday, August 23, 2010

The next day I sit down to ponder my weight problem. As I review the medications I am taking, I look more closely at Protonix. Protonix inhibits the production of acid that flows into my stomach. I decide this is the likely reason I am not gaining weight. With less acid, my stomach is unable to properly break down the food I am eating and, therefore, I am not getting its full nutritional value.

I will talk to Dr Hoagland on my next visit.

August 31, 2010

About a week later, I am back in Sharp Hospital for a procedure. Dr. Hoagland wants me to have a defibrillator (AICD) implanted into my chest as a precaution against heart failure or erratic rhythms. This is a surgery I had refused over the last eleven months, but, I finally caved in and the surgery is scheduled for today.

I enter the hospital in the morning, am prepped and taken to a lab for the procedure. The doctor makes a small incision high on the left side of my torso and slips the device underneath my chest muscle. I am returned to my room for the night.

For whatever reason, the aftermath of this surgery is extremely painful. After leaving the hospital in June, I was given a narcotic to use at home, yet, I never took a single dose. But this is different. I hope the pain will subside quickly as I will only be in the hospital overnight.

September 2010

September 1, 2010

I am released from Sharp but am still quite uncomfortable. I take the recommended dose of the narcotic but it doesn't seem to have any effect.

I try sleeping when I arrive home in the afternoon, but am unable due to the pain. During the night, I sleep no better. I will call the hospital in the morning.

September 2, 2010

I speak to Kristi, Dr. Hoagland's nurse practitioner, about my problem and she suggests I double the dose I am taking of the narcotic. I do and I finally feel relief. But it is at a price. Drugs such as these have side effects, mainly constipation. I know this and try to head off the problem with another pill to keep things moving but I am not successful.

September 3, 2010

I have to use more extreme measures to overcome the constipation and stop taking the narcotic. I happily discover the pain is mostly gone and all I now need is Tylenol.

It is odd touching my chest and feeling the lump underneath, but I guess no more so than seeing a cord coming out from my waist.

Tuesday, September 14, 2010

Almost two weeks later, I have my regular appointment with Dr. Hoagland. I have been suffering from rather severe headaches and don't know why. I rarely have headaches, and these are especially painful and persistent.

Kristi enters the room and introduces me to Leslie, another of the nurse practitioners working at the San Diego Cardiac Center. Leslie was on maternity leave when I was in the hospital in June. Like almost everyone I encountered through this ordeal, Leslie is a gem. She and Kristi both take good care of me over the coming months. Leslie also later helps me through a very difficult time dealing with my disability insurance payments.

Kristi comes in to do her evaluation and I tell her of my problem. She takes my vitals and tells me my blood pressure is quite high.

"How is this possible?" I ask. "Doesn't the pump maintain a constant speed?"

"Yes, it does. But your heart is now competing with the pump. Your heart appears to be healing," she tells me.

I am stunned. Not only do I once again have a pulse which can be felt at my wrist, it is also possible to take my blood pressure the usual way, with a pressure cuff and a stethoscope.

"So what's next for me?" I ask.

"We can put you on the heart transplant list, you can keep the pump for the rest of your life or, considering your progress, there is the possibility you will get well enough to someday have it removed," she replies.

Healed? Removed? Is she joking? What will Dr. Hoagland have to say?

When Dr. Hoagland finishes his usual exam he too gives me encouraging words regarding my progress. I know I can't get ahead of myself, but after such a nightmarish twelve months, this is welcome news.

I am doing almost everything possible to get well under the direction of Drs. Hoagland and Filidei. But the one thing I am not yet doing is exercising. It is the next thing on my "to do" list.

I also ask Dr. Hoagland if I can discontinue taking the Protonix and he agrees. Once off the drug, I gain almost ten pounds in less than two weeks. I am on my way.

Thursday, September 23, 2010

It is unreasonable for me to attend cardiac rehab in San Diego because of the distance. So, I contact Dr. Michaels about starting cardiac rehab in Mission Viejo. A stress test is scheduled for today to determine where the nurses in rehab will start my treatment.

I am connected to a variety of leads and put on a treadmill. The test will last a maximum of six minutes. I start walking slowly and after about three or four minutes they increase the speed slightly. I can make it no longer than about four minutes. I am exhausted and I am also rather embarrassed. Once again, my mind has decided I am stronger and healthier than is actually the case.

I will start on Monday at the rehab clinic in the hospital complex.

Monday, September 27, 2010

Today is my first day of Cardiac Rehab. Carol is the nurse in charge of the unit. With her are Elaine, Cindy and Terry. I begin by connecting myself to a telemetry device which monitors my heart rate and sends the information to a computer at the nurses' desk in the middle of the room.

The center is much like a small gym. There are treadmills, elliptical devices and a few other fitness machines, including free weights. I am started on a very slow program and monitored closely.

My schedule is to come to the center three times a week. The length of time and level of difficulty will be increased as warranted.

I am the only LVAD patient in rehab and am a bit of a novelty. But then, this is true almost anywhere I go. Everyone in the medical profession wants to break out their stethoscope and listen to my chest to hear the hum of the pump.

My order for rehab will last approximately four months. At that time I will need to look for another avenue for exercise. For now, this is exactly the right place for me.

I strongly recommend to anyone having this type of surgery to get into rehab as soon as your doctor permits. It is extremely beneficial to both your body and to your outlook.

October 2010

Wednesday, October 6, 2010

I go for my regular appointment with Dr. Michaels, my cardiologist in Mission Viejo. I am still excited about my last meeting with Dr. Hoagland, my cardiologist in San Diego and Sharp Hospital, and the optimistic news he gave me about the possibility of having the LVAD removed at some point in the future.

Dr. Michaels enters the examination room and before he has done any assessment I ask him, "Are you in contact with my doctors in San Diego?"

He says he does receive some updates from them.

"Have you heard they are thinking it may be possible in the near future to remove the device because my heart is healing?"

He looks blankly at me for a moment or two and replies, "Don't get your hopes up."

I am not a particularly aggressive person but I almost reach forward, grab him by his collar, yank him toward me and say, "You go to hell!" He has not examined me, I tell myself, knows nothing about the current condition of my heart, does not know why Dr. Hoagland sees this option as a possibility, but what he does know, again for absolute certainty, is that I "shouldn't get my hopes up."

This is the last time I see Dr. Michaels. I want to get well and I know I can't get there being around anyone who seems to revel in my being sick.

I call Dr. Hoagland's office and tell them I will be coming down monthly for my appointments; I will no longer see my cardiologist in Orange County.

Tuesday, October 19, 2010

Everything seems to be on track. I am feeling better, am making good progress in cardiac rehab, am taking fewer naps in the afternoon, and in general am feeling great.

Amazingly, after the massive exodus of my hair follicles in July, they are returning. What is a surprise, though, is my normally straight hair now has very distinctive waves running throughout. I don't know if it is a temporary or permanent change. But for now, I think it is kind of cool.

Susan, my friend and temporary roommate and caregiver, finds a new place to live and plans to move at the end of October. I knew her stay was temporary from the very beginning, yet I am also very sad at the thought of her leaving. I don't actually need the "care" aspect of her living with me, but it is nice not being alone. But it is time; she is ready and it is back to just me and my little dog.

Susan continues to help and support me. I will always cherish her friendship and kindness, especially during this time in my life when I needed her the most.

December 2010

Tuesday, December 7, 2010

Today is my regular appointment with Dr. Hoagland. In addition to the usual routine, I have an echocardiogram to check my progress. An echocardiogram is a non-invasive view of the heart, much like an ultrasound used to look at a fetus in its mother's uterus. Echocardiograms provide a wealth of information about the performance of the heart and are able to show possible problems with valves, performance of each chamber, and from it they are able to calculate the ejection fraction: the percent of blood expelled from the heart chamber with each beat.

After the test, I walk to the office area and wait to meet with Kristi, Dr. Hoagland's nurse practitioner, and Dr. Hoagland. Before surgery, my ejection fraction was below twenty. A normal heart has an ejection fraction of sixty or higher. Since my heart was unable to pump enough blood to meet the demands of my body, it kept pumping harder and, therefore, kept getting bigger.

Six months after surgery, my ejection fraction has risen to thirty-five, almost a 100% increase in output. Dr. Hoagland is pleased with the improvement and tells me we will repeat the test in March, three months from now. Until then, I need to keep doing what I am doing and hopefully continue to get better.

I ask him, "What is the target number? When will you consider removing the device?"

He tells me my ejection fraction needs to be above fifty before we can move ahead.

Fifty is now my goal.

I am elated. I leave the office and begin driving the seventy-five miles up the coast to my home in Aliso Viejo. I stop in Carlsbad for lunch at a small French bistro I know. The food is always good, but today it tastes just a little bit better.

February 2011

Friday, February 11, 2011

It has been about four months since I started cardiac rehab and today is my last day. The nurses send me off with best wishes. Carol, the head nurse in rehab, tells me she is convinced I will one day have the LVAD removed. I know how good the time has been for me in rehab and also know I have to keep exercising.

I drive directly from the hospital complex to a 24-Hour Fitness gym near my home. I sign up to start Monday morning.

Monday, February 14, 2011

I wake early, take Honey for her walk, feed her and leave for the gym. This will now be my new routine, five days a week.

At the gym, I start with the treadmill and walk briskly for about fifteen minutes. At the pace I set, this means I walk the equivalent of about one mile. From the treadmill I go to the weight machines and put together a routine to tone the rest of my body.

Most of the treadmills face a wall mirror. Seeing myself walking while wearing my equipment bag makes me laugh. I wonder what everyone must think.

"What is in that damn bag that is so valuable he can't leave it at home or in his car?"

But, most people at the gym pretty much keep to themselves and no one asks.

Since going off the Protonix in September, my weight has returned to normal. I now weigh 220 pounds, only ten pounds less than when this ordeal started. Friends are no longer looking at me with pity, and that feels good as well.

Many of the books I have read since falling ill (such as "Overcoming Thyroid Disorders" by Dr. David Brownstein and "Hypothyroidism: Type 2" by Dr. Mark Starr) refer to studies conducted by Dr. Broda Barnes and his book, "Solved: The Riddle of Heart Attacks." I begin searching for the book to read it. This is easier said than done. The book is out of print and any used copy I find is outrageously priced.

I eventually discover the Broda Barnes Foundation website and learn I can buy a copy of the book in a ring binder. I order it and look forward to receiving and reading this clearly influential work.

March 2011

Wednesday, March 16, 2011

Susan, my temporary roommate after I returned to my home last July, agrees to go with me to my appointment with Dr. Hoagland in San Diego. I am quite hopeful about the results of my echocardiogram today and want the moral support. After my gains in my ejection fraction of last year, I actually think I might have already reached an ejection fraction of fifty.

It is an odd day in the doctor's office. They are short an echocardiogram technician so my appointment is delayed. The technician I have is new and the test takes longer than usual. Afterward I realize I am scheduled not with Dr. Hoagland but with a different cardiologist. Normally I wouldn't mind, but today especially, I want my regular "team."

My ejection fraction is forty. I leave the office telling myself I am still moving in the right direction and this is not a setback. I got ahead of myself and know I need to calm down and get back to work. I am fine, my heart is still improving and I have no reason to be disappointed.

Thursday, March 17, 2011

After receiving and quickly reading the book by Dr. Barnes, I set an appointment for today with Dr. Filidei, my holistic doctor in Newport Beach. The book has raised further questions about the path I am currently taking to heal myself (I describe "my path" in detail in the final section of this book), this being addressing the hypothyroidism by taking Armour Thyroid. I question whether or not I am taking a high enough dose of the medication. I walk in, armed with books, printouts and so forth, much as I did over a year ago when seeing Dr. Michaels, my cardiologist in Mission Viejo. But Dr. Filidei is not Dr. Michaels in any sense.

I ask if he will write me an order for further blood tests as well as make adjustments to my medications, specifically the Armour Thyroid. I justify my requests based on what I have read in Dr. Barnes' book.

Dr. Filidei listens patiently and makes his counter proposal. He agrees to give me an order for the blood test but also wants me to conduct a seven-day basal body temperature test at home. After that time, I am to return and he will review the results of both. Dr. Filidei will then determine how to proceed.

A most pleasant difference in attitude from Dr. Michaels.

Friday, March 25, 2011

Dr. Filidei calls me at home with the blood test results and I relay to him my findings from the basal body temperature test. He agrees to increase my dose of Armour Thyroid and tells me to also increase my dose of human growth hormone.

My next echocardiogram is scheduled for June, almost three months from today. There is nothing more I can do but continue with my medications, my diet (these are explained in detail in Part III of this book), and my daily exercise.

One thing I need to point out. Although I have health insurance, much of what I am taking is not covered. My monthly costs of drug co-pays, drugs not covered by insurance and nutrients, run me about $800 with the majority of that cost being human growth hormone. It is and has been a major financial commitment but one I deem worthwhile. I think the results speak for themselves.

June 2011

Saturday, June 3, 2011

Three months later it is my grand-niece Natalie's second birthday celebration. It is hard to believe all that has happened this past year. On her first birthday I was little more than an old, sick man, slowly dying. It was difficult for me to even hold her while sitting. Today, I am my old self and able to enjoy being with her and my family. Unlike last year, I no longer wonder if today will be the last time I see them.

Monday, June 13, 2011

A week later at the gym, I think about tomorrow and my echocardiogram. I so want to hit the magic number of fifty for my ejection fraction but I remind myself that anything higher than March's number of forty is still progress.

My gym workouts have dramatically improved. I now walk on the treadmill for about twenty to twenty-five minutes at slightly higher than four miles per hour. After the treadmill I spend about thirty-five minutes working out with the machines and free weights.

I feel great and now want to get rid of the seven-pound bag of batteries I carry on my left shoulder. I especially want to swim again and take a real shower. I think briefly about being outside at the pool or in the gym locker room with my torso looking like something out of a Frankenstein movie, but I don't care. I want to feel the sensation of cool water once again gliding across my bare skin.

Yes, in the end it really is the simple pleasures in life that are most important.

Tuesday, June 14, 2011

I drive myself to San Diego today. I don't want to make a big deal out of this appointment by bringing my friend Susan with me. If the results of my ejection fraction are less than fifty, I want to be upbeat, as best I can, and get back to work on my health.

I go to the lab for the echocardiogram and try to see if I can read the technician's face, as if somehow her expression will tell me my current ejection fraction. Of course, this is silly, but no more so than anything else I have done over the last eighteen months. After the test, I dress and walk downstairs to Dr. Hoagland's office and sit down to wait.

Kristi, Dr. Hoagland's nurse practitioner, calls for me and we enter the examination room. Kristi does her usual assessment and we review my medications. She then leaves to get Dr. Hoagland.

Dr. Hoagland and Kristi enter the room together. Dr. Hoagland has the oddest expression on his face, one I have never seen before. I can't tell if he is about to deliver really good news or really bad news. He turns and breaks out in a smile.

He says, "Are you ready to come in and have the pump removed? Your ejection fraction is fifty."

I can't hold back the tears.

Kristi comes over and puts her arm around me saying, "This is what you have been working toward. Why are you crying?"

Dr. Hoagland also misinterprets my emotions and says, "I know, it's kind of scary to go back into surgery, but everything will work out just fine."

"This isn't about being afraid." I say. "You have to understand that for the last eighteen months my entire life has been focused on getting well. It has been as if I have been carrying around this heavy bag and now suddenly, you've told me I can set it down. I feel relief, joy and gratitude."

We discuss the next steps and I leave the office.

Wednesday, June 15, 2011

I am still walking on a cloud from yesterday's news. The device will finally be removed. It is incredible. Everything I have done has paid off. I still have several wickets to pass through before surgery, but I am on my way.

Now my biggest problem is patience.

Thursday, June 16, 2011

Every Thursday morning the transplant committee meets to discuss the cases before them. Today the members discuss how to proceed with my case. I have been given several possible scenarios by the staff, such as slowing down the speed of the pump over several weeks or entering the hospital and have the pumped slowed to a complete stop while they closely monitor me. But the decisions today will set my course.

It is decided I will come in on July 6 and have the speed of the pump reduced. This is to see if my heart will properly compensate for the loss of assistance from the LVAD.

July 2011

Wednesday July 6, 2011

Susan, my friend and now ex-roommate for the three months after I returned home from the hospital last year, picks me up at 9:15 a.m. and we drive to Sharp Hospital. I will have another echocardiogram; but this time, during the examination, Suzanne, one of the LVAD nurses, will begin slowing the pump's speed. My LVAD is currently set at a rate of 9200 revolutions per minute and has been at that level since being implanted.

As the technician begins to get readings on my heart, Suzanne starts to slow the speed by 200 rpm at a time. After each reduction they watch my heart to see how it responds. Both seem quite happy with the results, and they finally settle on a speed of 8400 rpm.

"We've only removed three of these devices before and each patient did well after its removal," says Suzanne. "I will tell you that your heart looks better than any of the others. You should do very well."

I dress, pack up my equipment, find Susan and we walk to the parking structure. Just before reaching the elevator I feel a bit lightheaded. I immediately turn around and walk back into the hospital and find Suzanne in the hall. I tell her what I am feeling.

She says, "We've just been talking about this and you are probably a little freaked out. Don't worry, you're fine. Go out and get lunch somewhere close and see how you feel. Come back if you feel the need."

Susan and I go to a taco stand not far from the hospital. I seem to feel better after getting some food and we head for home. About ten miles into the journey I feel as if I can't concentrate on the road and pull over and ask Susan to drive the rest of the way. Once home, I take a nap.

From then on, I feel fine. My heart is compensating for the lower pump speed.

Thursday July 7, 2011

I go to the gym for my morning workout. I am a bit concerned about how my heart will respond under the stress of exercise. I first consider doing a lighter routine but instead go forward as if nothing has happened.

I leave the gym feeling no different than two days before. Everything seems to be going quite well.

Wednesday July 13, 2011

I drive myself to Sharp Hospital for a follow-up echocardiogram after the slowing of the pump, one week ago. For this visit, Marcia, also an LVAD nurse who works with Suzanne, is with me to monitor the test. Both Marcia and the technician are quite pleased with the results and see nothing that might interfere with the removal of the device. In addition to the echo, I also have a CT scan of my chest. This is for Dr. Adamson, the surgeon, for reference during the actual surgery to remove the LVAD.

After both tests, I go with Marcia to their office in Sharp Hospital and wait to meet with Dr. Adamson who wants to see me prior to surgery the following week. We chat briefly and the date for surgery is set for Friday, July 22. It is a rather awkward date as Dr. Hoagland will be out of town the 21st through the 24th, Dr. Hoagland's nurse practitioners, Leslie and Kristi, will be gone the entire week, and Dr. Adamson will be leaving on vacation on the 23rd. After seeing this journey through with the entire team I feel a little as if I am cheating on them by not proceeding on a day on which everyone can be present. But, they will all be back on the following Monday, and at this point, I don't want to wait any longer than necessary.

So, I am scheduled to enter the hospital on Wednesday, July 20, for surgery on Friday, July 22.

Tuesday, July 19, 2011

I need to complete a pre-surgery task. I drive to San Bernardino taking my dog, Honey, to my cousin Cindy's house. Cindy took care of Honey while I was in Sharp the prior year. I have to say I am a little hesitant dropping her off. Last year, Honey liked staying with Cindy so much she was a little unsure about coming home with me. But, at least I know Cindy will take good care of my little girl and that is what is most important.

Wednesday, July 20, 2011

Susan picks me and my equipment up at 7:45 a.m., and we head down the coast.

I had some trouble sleeping the night before, from a mix of excitement and anxiety. As much as I want the device removed I also know I am once again facing major surgery. I wonder how I will react this time. Will I be as terrified on Friday morning as I was a little over a year ago? Or will I act calmly, like a seasoned pro? Only time will tell.

After registering at the hospital, I am given my room number and a volunteer comes to escort me. As we pass the nurse's desk, Laura, the angel of a nurse who helped me the prior year, looks up at me and smiles. She comes around the desk and gives me a hug. She and the entire staff are excited for me and I am happy to see them. She apologizes for my room, since it is on the side of the hospital without a view.

"I'll do what I can to get you moved. Something should open up soon," she promises.

I get to the room, change into the most unflattering piece of clothing ever made and settle into bed for the string of tests I know will be coming. But, other than a minor blood test, I am pretty much left alone.

Shortly after noon, the echocardiogram technician wheels in her machine and starts setting up for what I believe will be the last time. She measures all parameters while I briefly drift off from lack of sleep the night before. As she finishes, both Dr. Hoagland and Dr. Adamson come into my room to view the results.

After seeing the replay of the test Dr. Adamson looks down at me and says, "You have nothing to worry about. Your heart looks basically normal, as if none of this had ever happened. You'll do great."

That afternoon, true to her word, Laura finds me a room on the "view" side of the hospital and I move into my deluxe suite.

Thursday, July 21, 2011

It is a day of mostly waiting. There are few pre-surgery events except for a bath and a wipe-down with sterile solutions. Also there is a rather nasty process of spreading a salve onto a Q-tip and swabbing it in my nose. Very unpleasant.

After everything I have read, I am more aware of the food served in hospitals and how it lacks the nutrients our bodies need, especially under the stress of sickness or surgery. One tray I receive is mostly carbohydrates: steamed vegetables, fruit, macaroni and cheese, with only a few, tiny pieces of chicken for protein. I want raw, whole milk to drink, but am unable to arrange having it in the hospital. I decide I will ask visiting friends to bring food when they come to see me. That way I can get the balance of nutrition I have been eating at home.

Marcia comes by and asks if I am willing to talk to a fifty-nine-year-old patient in medical ICU about the LVAD. He is on the list for a heart transplant but has been in and out of the hospital for several months while waiting. They proposed the LVAD to him but he is still unsure. He asked if he could speak to someone who has the device and has lived with it for a while. With nothing in particular to do, I am more than happy to get out of my room and meet him.

We have a pleasant chat and I tell him of my experience with the pump. I encourage him to go forward with the implant because I know how badly he must have been feeling over the last several months. I tell him the pump will greatly improve his quality of life and from what I have been told earlier, am confident he can still proceed with the transplant if he chooses. His nurse then enters his room, that being the sign for me to leave.

About 2:30 p.m., Kevin arrives from Dallas to stay with me during the surgery and for several days after. It is good to see him and good to have someone to talk to. I must say, being in the hospital when you feel great is very boring. You have no need to rest, relax, take it easy, or anything else.

About 5:30 p.m., my day nurse, Leah, comes in with something in her hand and a rather wry smile on her face.

"Mr. Martin, we have to take the next step in preparing you for surgery."

My eyes drift down to her hand, trying to determine what she must be holding. She doesn't make me wait long. It is a suppository. With a sigh of resignation I roll to my side and she performs the unpleasant deed.

Anissa is my nurse that evening. Although I am quite calm I feel sure I will not sleep well and ask for something to help me get through the night. She brings me an Ambien, which I take, and that pretty much ends the day for me.

Friday, July 22, 2011

I wake on my own at 4:30 am. Already there is movement outside my room. I thought I might be filled with panic but I am remarkably calm.

Anissa comes in with the nurse's assistant, both armed with electric razors. "We have to shave your entire body, neck down."

Making probably my final attempt at some level of modesty I ask, "Isn't there a male nurse available to do this?"

"No, there isn't."

So, off with my gown and the shaving games begin. At my height, it is a lot of real estate to cover. When finished, I realize they have only shaved the front of my legs.

"No, no, if you are going to shave my legs, you have to do a complete job."

They oblige and my body now looks as if I am ten years old. Well, not quite, but at least the same level of body hair.

They give me one last antiseptic bath, one more dose of the nose gel and I am ready to go. The gel in my nose is to prevent the MRSA virus, something that concerns every hospital. Once it takes hold in a patient, it can easily spread to others and they do their best to ensure this does not happen. MRSA is also resistant to treatment.

They wheel me out of my room and on to the SPA. With a name like SPA, you think of a quiet, soothing, pleasant retreat. Nope, SPA stands for Surgery Procedure Area. There is absolutely nothing soothing about it. It is basically a staging area before entering an operating room. I chat with the nurse and with Marcia while waiting.

One interesting thing about surgeries and other major, invasive procedures, they bring you paperwork to sign right before they wheel you in. There is no real chance to read what you are signing or even ponder what might lie ahead. It is a clever way to avoid protests from patients. This seems to be the procedure in all hospitals.

It is time. I am wheeled into the operating room fully aware of what is happening. I am asked to move from the gurney onto the operating table. So this is what an operating room really looks like, I tell myself.

The circulating nurse comes over and she, Marcia, and I begin to talk. An x-ray of my chest is hanging on the wall and both of them comment how good everything looks. They point out to me various landmarks on the film, such as my heart, my stomach, the LVAD, and tell me what they are.

The anesthesiologist introduces himself and says, "I'm going to give you something to help you relax."

We obviously have different definitions of the word "relax" because whatever he gives me completely knocks me out. I don't even get the chance to count backwards from one hundred.

When I open my eyes three hours later something inside of me already knows that things have not gone as planned.

Marcia is standing over me. Even though I am still somewhat under the influence I can still comprehend what she is saying. "The surgery didn't happen. We ran into a problem with a vein in your neck. As an alternate approach we decided to use the vein below your heart. The problem is that you have an implanted filter and it prevents access. They decided to remove the filter but couldn't because they did not have the necessary instrument. I am so sorry."

I was shaved, scrubbed and anesthetized for nothing.

Maybe because I still have anesthesia running through my veins, I take the news very calmly. I'd like to say I'm the type of guy who rolls with the punches and never gets upset, but this is far from the truth. By the following day, though, I will realize how disappointed I truly am.

For now, they take me back to my room. Everyone, even nurses and staff I've never met are giving me their regrets.

I tell Kevin, "Drive to the taco stand down the street and get me a mega-burrito. I'm hungry and I need something to let me down easy."

Even under the last traces of anesthesia that burrito tastes oh, so good.

That evening when the nursing shift changes, I am sitting on the couch in my hospital room. Anissa is once again my night nurse. She comes in, sits down next to me and gives me a hug, telling me how sorry she is that the surgery was aborted.

It isn't quite the same as waking up without the LVAD, but I must admit, it is a very nice hug.

Saturday, July 23, 2011

The morning mood in the unit is rather somber. I think everyone wants to forget the prior day's events. I am taken for a chest x-ray but no other tests are run. Suzanne comes to my room and tells me I will probably come back the week of August 1 to have the IVC filter removed and then back for surgery on August 11.

I pack up my stuff, am discharged, and Kevin drives me home, still a little numb from the shock of the prior three days.

Tuesday, July 26, 2011

Only three days later, the scheduling department at Sharp Hospital calls, wanting to set a time for the IVC filter removal the next day.

The next day? I ask myself. Has the instrument arrived so quickly? I tell the woman I don't think it is possible for me to have the procedure the next day as I am taking the blood thinner Coumadin.

This causes her to pause and she tells me she will call back. She does and says the procedure is re-scheduled for Friday.

After we hang up, I still think it is odd about the instrument arriving so soon. So, I call Suzanne, one of the LVAD nurses, and tell her the procedure is set for Friday. She doesn't seem to be too surprised, so I mistakenly assume that I alone am uneasy about how quickly everything is moving.

In retrospect, I should have asked to speak to the doctor performing the filter removal.

I should have asked, "Have you seen the instrument? Have you held it in your hands? Is it truly the one you need?"

Instead, I trust the machinery that is a hospital and begin making arrangements to return to Sharp on Friday.

Friday July 29, 2011

We leave my home at 6:15 a.m. Once again, my friend Susan offers to drive down with me, spend the day waiting and then drive me home.

After arriving at the hospital and going to registration I am escorted to an area near the SPA. It is a series of curtained-off beds with patients being prepared for one procedure or another. After once again depositing my shoes and clothes in the courtesy bag, a nurse comes in and starts the IV. She has to try twice to actually make it happen. I think my veins are finally protesting from the abuse they have taken over the last two years. With the IV finally in place, what next but more paperwork to sign. It is quite difficult to sign anything when there is a large needle stuck in a vein in your hand. But, I do the best I can.

Another nurse then walks in with an electric razor and says, "I need to shave your groin."

"It's unnecessary," I reply, "There's nothing left to shave. It was all removed last week."

Not believing me, she lifts the sheet and we both observe my prepubescent-looking genital area. Not leaving without performing some task, she takes cloths infused with an antiseptic liquid and begins vigorously wiping the entire area.

I smile and think about all those episodes of "Law & Order" when someone is asked if they were touched inappropriately. I ask myself, I wonder if this qualifies.

After a short wait, someone from the transport department comes to take me to the room in which the procedure will be performed. We get to the door and discover the patient before me is not yet finished. So they wheel me into a smaller waiting area for what they say will only be five or ten minutes.

Ten minutes later, a nurse comes in to give me the news. "We don't have the instrument, it's not here. But, there is a delivery coming shortly, it may be in that package. We will also call around to other hospitals nearby to see if we can borrow one from them."

Another fifteen minutes passes and the same nurse comes into the room saying, "We have the instrument. You'll have to wait another fifteen or twenty minutes because we let the next scheduled patient go ahead of you. But everything is going to be fine."

I wait and I wait some more. Then the doctor who will be performing the procedure comes into the room.

He says, "I don't know why anyone scheduled you for today. The instrument doesn't even exist. It has to be custom built. There is no way it could have been made and delivered in so short a time. It will probably take four to eight weeks from when it was ordered on July 22."

I am fortunate to have a mechanism as part of my makeup that almost completely shuts me down when I get very, very angry. As I listen to the doctor and then the nurse review the situation, all I can do is silently stare at them. How on earth could someone, everyone, screw up this badly? Part of me wants to start yelling at anyone within earshot but part of me also knows better. I need to keep my mouth shut for the moment and find out later what went wrong. I also still need these people, and I see no good reason to get everyone mad at me.

I am angry, upset and disappointed. Maybe the frustration of this and the prior week's events hits me all at once. I say little to anyone. I just want to get dressed and leave. I return to the prep area, get back into my clothes and along with Susan, leave the hospital.

When things go wrong in my life, my "cure" is to go out for a nice lunch. We drive to La Jolla to one of my favorite places in the

San Diego area called Tapenade. We have a wonderful lunch, a glass or two of wine and suddenly, life looks a little bit better.

I pay the bill and keep the receipt. I will turn it over to someone, someday for reimbursement. I think it is the least they can do for me.

August 2011

Wednesday, August 10, 2011

A week later, I am watching television when my phone rings about 10:00 a.m.

"Mr. Martin? It's Sharp Hospital. Where are you? Are you coming in?"

Oh no, I think, did I forget to write something down in my calendar? What did I miss? I'm usually good about these kinds of thing.

"Come in for what exactly?" I ask.

"I don't know," she tells me. "We have a bed reserved for you on the cardiac floor. You were supposed to check into the hospital at 9:00 a.m."

"No, no, that was all postponed. I was to have surgery tomorrow but it was cancelled."

"Who cancelled it?" she asks.

"I don't know who would be in charge of that," I reply. "But I can give you a list of names to start calling."

Monday, August 29, 2011

I call Marcia, an LVAD nurse who works with Suzanne, to see if someone can contact the manufacturer of the instrument and check on its status. I want to be sure things are actually moving forward.

When she answers the phone, I identify myself.

She begins to chuckle. "Were your ears burning? We were just talking about you. We have an update on the status of the instrument."

Then she tells me, "The instrument has been built and is undergoing sterilization. It will soon be shipped and should arrive at

Sharp by September 9. So, the first procedure will probably be scheduled for the week of September 12 and the LVAD removal surgery for the week of September 19." She also says, "After what happened last month, we don't want to schedule anything until we have the instrument in hand. But, we also need to reserve space on the calendars of the two doctors who will be handling these cases."

So, if everything goes as planned, I will be LVAD-free in about three and a half weeks.

I'll bring the champagne if someone else brings the balloons and party hats!

Wednesday, August 31, 2011

Marcia calls with great glee in her voice to tell me the instrument has arrived.

The date is set for Wednesday, September 7 at 9:00 a.m. for the removal of the IVC filter. It is a one-day, outpatient procedure and will take me one step closer to life without the LVAD.

September 2011

Thursday, September 1, 2011

I receive more good news from San Diego. The date of my surgery is set for Thursday, the fifteenth. I will enter Sharp Hospital on the fourteenth in preparation.

Hopefully this time I will come home *sans* LVAD.

Wednesday, September 7, 2011

My friend Jay drives me to San Diego this morning, leaving my house at 5:45 a.m. We arrive at the hospital at 7:00 a.m., I check in and am escorted to the SPA for the same preparations as three weeks earlier.

Unlike my prior visit, the IVC filter is successfully removed. Two catheters are used for the retrieval, one entering from my neck and the other from my groin. From what I am told, it was wedged in rather tightly and it takes quite some time to pry out. What normally is a thirty-minute procedure turns into a two hour mini-marathon. I understand the radiologist did a "happy dance" in the lab after successfully extracting the long-legged filter. The deed is done and I am one major step closer to having reverse LVAD surgery.

I also learn that "one percent" is now "two percent." Two percent of LVAD patients worldwide are able to have the device removed, returning to life without needing a heart transplant.

Pretty exciting stuff, I think.

Wednesday September 14, 2010

Jay picks me up and drives me to Sharp Hospital. He drops me off with all of my equipment, the same stuff which won't be returning home with me. I feel great! Now I just have to get through the next few days of surgery and recovery.

They take me up to the fifth floor to my room, and I immediately start asking for my nursing friends. I'm saddened to find out that several of them no longer work at the hospital.

Thursday, September 15, 2010

It's 4:30 a.m. and it is time to head to surgery. I have already been shaved and swabbed sterile. My skin has a lovely cherry hue to it from the antiseptic solution they used to scrub my body. I am taken down to the SPA area and meet with the circulating nurse and my surgeon. Suzanne, my LVAD nurse buddy, is there to meet me. Much like in July, I'm surprised at how calm I am.

I am wheeled into the O.R. and the gurney is brought up next to the Operating table. I am told to move over onto it. It is unbelievably narrow. Inserts are put into the sides of the table to support my arms. But this moving myself from the gurney to the procedure tables is getting old. It somehow makes me think of a condemned man in prison being asked to start his own IV before the necessary injections are made.

I don't remember the anesthesiologist talking to me or giving me anything. I just know that suddenly I am out.

I also don't remember waking up this time. But I am back in the SPA with everyone keeping a close eye on me. I am then transferred to surgical ICU. I ask for certain nurses that I remember from last year. It is like old home week as they all pour in wishing me well. I cannot say enough good about the nursing staff at Sharp. Everyone is excited about my surgery, this is a really big deal and I think they are genuinely excited it was me who had the surgery.

When you have surgery as major as an LVAD implant, I think it is the Surgical ICU staff with whom you form the strongest bonds. You can't function hour to hour without them. You realize just how helpless a small child must feel and how dependent they are upon adults and why they cry so hard for their mommies and daddies when they are afraid. If I thought I could have gotten picked up and rocked, I probably would have started crying loudly as well.

As the hours pass in ICU, I realize that the staff is becoming quite concerned about me. I don't realize at the time just how badly things are going for me since I don't feel all that sick. The first minor nightmare is that they begin talking of reinserting the breathing tube while I am awake. This is something I know for great certainty, I don't want to happen.

They then decide they must reinsert the catheter. Again, I think of crying loudly, but know it will get me nowhere. Having a catheter inserted is one of the most uncomfortable things I've ever endured. They take the plastic tube and shove it down your urethra until it breaks through into your bladder. Your entire body shudders as it happens. I could only moan faintly, although I did think about screaming for a moment, to let everyone in the unit know that things can always be worse for them. The nurse then periodically had to check the tubing from the catheter and the flow of urine. About every thirty minutes or so she would come by, lift the bottom of my gown and stare quizzically at her prior handiwork. From my perspective, it seemed she was just "checking out the goods." I kept wondering, does it look ok? Is it green? Is it just really mad at you for inserting the tube? After this happened four or five times she came over and said, "We need to do some maintenance on the catheter, would you be more comfortable if a male nurse took care of this?" I would have been more comfortable if a male nurse had taken care of this three hours earlier. At this point, I no longer cared.

With the catheter now in place, they begin spraying a painkiller down my nose and my throat. It is very unpleasant. They then tip me back and insert a tube down my throat into my lungs to get a sample of the phlegm that is there. They are quite concerned I have pneumonia but they need to know the exact form so they can treat it properly. That task out of the way, I'm now looking forward to a break in activities. I have two drainage tubes coming out of my chest and have been told another procedure will be performed later that night.

The sac around my heart has become filled with fluid and is placing pressure on my heart. So, they go in through my groin and run a tube up to my heart and place this new drain to the sac. More shaving, more pain meds, more of everything.

I return to the room around midnight and try to relax and leave the last two days behind me. They also start me on CPap treatments. They cover my mouth with an oxygen mask type device that blows air into my lungs. It is more than simply uncomfortable, and it completely dries out my mouth. I have to have these sessions about once every couple of hours for one hour at a time. They are trying to get me well to avoid reinserting the breathing tube. That is the carrot they dangle in front of me. I'm more than happy to cooperate. Well, I'm not actually happy, I just don't want any more heavy drugs pumped into me. They also determine the best treatment for the pneumonia and add the antibiotics to my IV.

Sunday, September 18, 2011

Dr. Hoagland, my cardiologist, comes in and tells me repeatedly how much better I look. "We thought we might lose you yesterday."

Now wouldn't that be ironic, I tell myself. I make it all this way only to die of pneumonia and not heart disease.

I am transferred out of ICU and back to the cardiac unit on the fifth floor.

I am now on the fast track of healing. They will probably take out the drainage tubes on Thursday, which means there is a chance I can go home on Friday.

Thursday, September 22, 2011

My nurse angel from last year is my nurse again today. Lisa walks in with her beautiful smile and I know this will be a good day all around.

My night nurse cleans me up and changes the dressings on my torso. Rip, rip, rip... For all the advances in non-stick glue, none seems to have filtered down to pharmaceuticals. The hair follicles on my torso constantly protest in spite of my best, earlier efforts at having everything shaved to avoid these uncomfortable confrontations.

They remove the first of the drains in my chest. The first one removed had been inserted into my side and went to my heart. It is the strangest sensation having one removed. Not painful, just odd. Breathing at the right times makes all the difference. A male and a female nurse practitioner come in and I tell them they will have to get Lisa before they can continue.

"Why," says the male, "Do you need her to hold your hand?"

"Damn straight I do!" I tell him.

Friday, September 23, 2011

I am discharged from the hospital and Susan brings me home. She decides to spend a couple of days with me, to keep an eye on my progress and be there if I need anything.

When I go up to bed, I am almost beside myself. With no bag across my shoulder, I can simply remove my shirt, and I don't need to sit down to accomplish the task. Whoosh! It's off. The weather has also turned much cooler and I slip under the sheet, blanket and heavy comforter. It feels so wonderful being back in my own bed that I begin to giggle, something I don't normally do.

Saturday, September 24, 2011

I get up this morning and put on a robe. I don't need to nor do I really even want to. I put one on because I *can* for the first time in 15 months. It feels great!!

Sunday, September 25, 2011

I go to Dr. Kennedy's wedding and have a great time. I even get up and dance. It feels great moving across the floor without that damn bag around my neck!!

Monday, September 26, 2011

Now it is all about getting back to a normal routine at home. I look at all of the things I really should be doing and feel a bit overwhelmed. I need to get back to the gym but, for some reason, I am a bit hesitant. I ask myself: What's next?

So, What is Next?

I wish I had known in September 2009 what I know now. I believe I could have made the necessary changes in my life and avoided surgery. But I also know that in June 2010, the LVAD was my only option.

The LVAD did not heal my heart but it did give my heart the *opportunity* to heal. The rest depended upon me and what path and action I took. The LVAD restored blood flow to all vital functions in my body and, therefore, as I changed my diet and took various nutrients and hormones, my heart could heal.

So now I can get my life back to "normal." Actually, I need a new definition for that word. While on disability, my entire department at work was laid off so I have no job to return to. Also, because my background is in software development and I have not worked in two years, I am considered "stale" and software companies are not usually interested in hiring those like me.

I have to redefine myself. I have to find a new path. But at least I have options and once again, this is no time to sit around and feel sorry for myself. I need to focus on my accomplishments over the last two years and act. Writing this book has been one such outlet.

Remember, "Hope is a good thing, maybe the best thing."

Part II

Taking Control – Your Health, Your Responsibility

"Unhappily too, this is the Dark Age of Medicine…"
— Henry G. Bieler, M.D.

Lessons Learned

This section covers what I have learned during this experience about my health and the health attitudes of others. Obviously, this section is not complete. I have read so many books about health and nutrition, it would be impossible to effectively summarize them in this book. You must understand the "why" behind the "what" you should be doing.

The two questions I have been asked most often since my surgery in June 2010 is "How has this changed you? What have you learned?"

I'm never quite sure how to interpret the questions. Do they mean have I learned something on a more spiritual or cosmic level? Are they asking if my goals in life have changed? Or do they mean something more basic such as: what was my life like with the LVAD?

One definite change is my view of others with illnesses and disabilities. When I used to enter a hospital or medical building prior to having the LVAD I used to simply walk by people confined to wheelchairs or struggling with other debilitating diseases, not fully noticing them. Now I actually see them. I see them and wonder about their lives and their daily routines. How do they bathe? How do they prepare meals? What adjustments did they have to make in their lives? How have they handled those changes? Will they get well?

The second and most important lesson learned is how critical a good attitude is to reaching wellness. I remember when I first returned to work in November 2009, shortly after I had been diagnosed with heart failure. I was about to walk over to the cafeteria to get some breakfast when my friend and coworker Stephen said, "Here, I'll get that for you, it's a long walk." I paused for a moment. It would be rather nice to be waited upon but I also realized I would be setting my own path at that very moment. Was I to be a victim, calling upon others to care for me? Or would I take the situation and reverse it? I chose the latter. I thanked Stephen for his offer but walked over and retrieved breakfast on my own.

In the first months after surgery I regularly compared my life to those in far worse situations than me. I had to remind myself that, with the exceptions of bathing and swimming, my life was pretty much as it had been two years earlier. I could move around freely, live alone, cook my meals, shop, walk my dog, and so forth. I had to focus on what I could do, not upon what I could not do. Don't misunderstand, I did cry a lot at first. I grieved over the part of my life I was losing. But it seemed that shortly after surgery, I knew it was time to buck up and move forward.

Sharp Hospital holds monthly LVAD support group meetings. I attended one and only one gathering. In general, the people attending were friendly and dealing well with living with the device. But when two people with a "poor me" attitude began speaking, I knew I had to leave.

I also remembered what my mother said to me as a child when I would whine and complain about how unfair life was. She would look up and say, "Get your shoes on. I'm taking you down to County Hospital where you can see children dying from cancer and then you can tell me how unfair your life really is!" I often drew upon her wisdom from the moment I began to feel that life had been unfair to me by giving me heart disease.

Kyle Maynard was born with no arms and no legs from the elbows and knees down. Instead of treating him as a victim, his parents expected the same from him as from their other children. He played baseball as a child and was later on the wrestling team in high school with a record of 35 wins and 16 losses. He has written a book, traveled, appeared on talk shows and does motivational speaking. How can I pity myself or complain because I merely carry around a satchel in the face of this man's experience?

I have always read and studied the effects of nutrition and diet on health. But my experience motivated me to investigate further and expand my knowledge. What I have learned during these last two years only further confirms what I have always known. Instead of merely accepting what I was told by the medical industry, I had to take responsibility for my own wellness. I needed to do my own research, to seek out the proper doctors and to make the necessary changes to my life to move toward optimal health.

I had already begun questioning the medical establishment while still in my teens. Our neighbor, Sid, had arthritis so badly he was barely able to walk. His doctor told him he would soon be confined to a wheelchair. They could treat the symptom of pain, but there was nothing they could do for the actual disease of arthritis. Sid decided he didn't want to live the rest of his life sitting down so he got the book, "Arthritis and Common Sense" by Dale Alexander. The book advocates dietary changes and taking large doses of cod liver oil daily. Sid followed Mr. Alexander's advice and within six months he was walking and playing eighteen holes of golf. When he told his doctor what he had done and the results, the doctor said, "That approach is not the reason you are well." The doctor, not surprisingly, had no other explanation and no interest in what Dale Alexander recommended in his book. But what the doctor did know, with complete certainty, was he could learn nothing from Dale Alexander about treating arthritis.

The human body is an amazing machine. When damaged, it heals; when stressed, it compensates; when fed garbage, it does its best to take what is good and eliminate what is bad. But like any piece of machinery, if it is consistently, over time, treated and maintained badly, it will shut down. In the case of the human body, this manifests itself as disease.

Basically all pharmaceutical drugs are synthetic, not natural and organic. If you continue to put something synthetic into your body, is it any wonder your body will begin breaking down? Is it any wonder that the long-term ingestion of one drug almost always leads to a second drug to counter a reaction to the first? The second drug leads to a third and the third to a fourth. All the while the patient becomes increasingly ill and debilitated. A close friend's elderly mother was on so many drugs she was no longer able to walk. A new doctor looked at the list and eliminated most of her medications. She now feels great and is again walking around her home and her garden.

To quote Dr. David Brownstein, "You cannot poison a crucial enzyme or block an important receptor in the body for the long term and expect a good result."

Although my mother raised me with knowledge of proper diet and nutrition, I learned and researched extensively on what our bodies actually need to cure disease and reach optimal health. One thing is certain, nutrient-dense foods are not served up in shrink-wrapped packages. The more foods are processed before reaching our stomachs, the less beneficial they are to our bodies.

I remember in the early 1980s when the cholesterol scare was reaching its peak. One food identified as hazardous to our health was eggs. But not to worry, there was a solution and it was called Egg Beaters, a processed egg product. I was appalled. Eggs are one of nature's most perfect and complete foods. They are rich in proteins, calcium, enzymes, vitamins and other minerals and this is especially true of eggs from organically fed, free-range chickens. But the medical establishment told us that something made in a laboratory was healthier than something from nature. Of course, several years later the story changed. "Hmmm… maybe eggs aren't all that bad for you. Hmmm… maybe it's yolks that are bad and the whites are good?" Or maybe it was all a load of crap designed to sell packaged, processed food products and drugs.

As I tell people what I have read and learned, some are receptive and some are not. I am challenging their belief systems and that challenge is not welcomed. More than one person said, "But who do I trust? There is so much information out there on both sides of an issue. How can I possibly know who is right?" What I found as I read book after book, was one side of the argument always emerged as more complete than the other. I rarely use web-based articles for information as they are often too brief, incomplete and the sources of the material are unclear. I started with one book by Dr. Brownstein and that set the tone and approach for the rest of my reading.

I would love to effectively condense the thirty or so books I have read on health and nutrition into one or two pithy pages, but that is simply not possible. My goal is to provide some of what I have learned along the way with their proper references and hope you, too, take responsibility for your own health and wellness. Knowledge truly is power.

Challenging the Medical Establishment

By taking your health into your own hands you will, at times, be forced to confront and challenge your doctor and the views of the medical establishment. You may even find, as I did, the need to leave certain doctors for others. This is clearly too big a challenge for many people. To avoid the issue, they tend to justify their actions by defending the very people keeping them in a state of illness.

"Have you gotten better? Are you cured?" I have asked people I know.

"No, but my doctor is the best internist/dermatologist/cardiologist, etc. in all of Orange County!" has been a common reply.

Or, they may say, "If what you are saying is true, why doesn't *my* doctor know about it?"

This attitude causes me to wonder why people believe their doctor and their doctor alone, knows absolutely everything that can possibly be known about their specific illness. But, the origin of that attitude often originates with the doctor himself.

As I read books by Drs. Brownstein, Starr, Murphree, and others, and began following their advice, I was scoffed at by many people, especially those working in the medical field.

"Is a second opinion generally a good idea when approaching illness?" I would ask.

"Well, of course, there's nothing wrong with that," they would reply.

"There is no question as to my diagnosis, the concern, now, is my treatment. Why is it acceptable for me to get a second opinion from a doctor while in his office but not from a book he has written?" would be my next question to them.

If two doctors disagree on my treatment, even if I visit both in their offices, at least one of the doctors must be wrong. Deciding on a course of treatment, then, becomes my responsibility. Instead of spending fifteen minutes in an office hearing a doctor's advice, I spent hours reading their books to fully understand their positions. I believe it was time well spent and necessary to understand one approach over another.

My cousin Anna began searching for an endocrinologist open to a more natural approach to thyroid disease. Not wanting to waste time setting appointments with various doctors, as I did, only to discover they would not provide the desired treatment, she asked my advice how to target the proper physician.

I thought about her question and told her to call their offices and simply ask if the doctor is open to prescribing Armour Thyroid instead of Synthroid should treatment be necessary. The reaction of those she called was shocking. In one case, the doctor himself came to the phone and began yelling and berating Anna for even asking the question. Yep, there's a doctor I never want to see.

For a complete explanation about thyroid disorders and proper treatment, please read, *Overcoming Thyroid Disorders* by Dr. David Brownstein. I will attempt to summarize some of the material below.

Let's get one thing said. I don't care who your doctor is or what he has accomplished, he is NOT God. I know it would be much easier if that were actually the case, but it is not. Your doctor works for you. Just because you ask questions, no burly bouncer is going to enter the room and toss you out the window. If that were true, I'd have a permanent layer of broken glass all over my body.

I am amazed at the arrogance of the medical community believing that they alone hold the cure to illness and disease. Do they honestly believe they are smarter than the miracle of God's creation or millions of years of evolution? Within their laboratories and with great hubris, they create and manufacture drugs our bodies have never encountered and have no idea exactly how to process. Diets are designed in complete opposition to our nature and then those following these plans are surprised when they fall ill.

We are bombarded with advertising from pharmaceutical companies encouraging us to take one drug or another. We have heard the health warnings so often we've become desensitized to their message. In one case, which I will discuss in a future chapter, the written caveat in the advertisement clearly states that the drug doesn't even work for what it is intended. Every third commercial on television is for a drug and every fourth for a law firm suing a pharmaceutical company for the dangerous, sometimes lethal, side effects of their FDA-approved products. Yet we remain hungry for more, and doctors accommodate us by prescribing one synthetic drug after another even while seeing that their patients are not getting well. And still more sadly, too often if a patient protests that their treatment is not working, they will be diagnosed as "depressed" and will be prescribed yet another drug.

Another protest I have heard is, "But this is science! Look at all the studies they've conducted. Do you actually think these companies would put these products on the market if they were dangerous or didn't work? I mean, the FDA has approved it!"

Pharmaceutical companies have created, tested and marketed many FDA-approved drugs that have later been pulled from the shelves because of the extreme danger they pose to patients. Sadly, all drugs have negative side effects over time, but doctors keep prescribing and we, as a people, keep popping pills, which amounts to little more than poison to our bodies.

One more observation regarding the "scientific" aspect of drugs and their testing. I know two people who work in the pharmaceutical industry. One conducts clinical trials on new medications and one works in statistics, the department that compiles and evaluates the results of the various studies. I have been shocked in the past at how few patients are actually used in many studies, and this leads me to question the validity of their findings. Even more disturbing is the comment from my friend in statistics, "I can made the numbers say whatever my company wants them to say." That doesn't sound like "science" to me.

What puzzles me most is those who will not even consider any benefit to a more natural approach to healing. It is as if they are completely gripped with fear over the possibilities of dietary changes and adding nutrients to their diet. Why are they so willing to consume prescription drugs, each listing a page or two of warnings and yet are so unwilling to try a natural approach? Warnings on a currently prescribed drug include: liver damage, suicidal tendencies, muscle aches, joint pain, cancer, heart failure, and even death. Each contains significant risks yet those risks are ignored because of the hope of a simple cure. The cure, of course, never comes because the treatments almost exclusively target symptoms, not underlying causes of disease. Natural treatments--much like eating more carrots, more broccoli, etc., or taking naturally occurring nutrients such as vitamins A or C--usually carry no such negative side effects.

I realize under critical circumstances we often turn our lives over to those who we believe can best help us. But most health issues do not require immediate, invasive treatment for us to survive. We usually have time to address our disease and seek alternate treatment long before the situation becomes critical. In fact, many natural approaches to healing can be done in conjunction with traditional Western medicine. I am a good example of this. If I had not had the LVAD implanted, I would likely have died. I did continue to take several commonly prescribed heart medications while, at the same time, taking a wide array of nutrients and other prescribed medications that would help my heart heal.

By not educating ourselves and taking action, we make a serious commitment to disease and chronic illness instead of taking the path of health and wellness. To me, it would seem to be a rather easy and obvious choice.

But no, "If it worked, my doctor would know about it."

The Fatalists

In my travels through Europe I coined a phrase I call "The French Salute." Too often when asking for assistance or requesting a favor, French clerks would look up at me, raise their palms to the sky, shrug their shoulders and say, "Monsieur, there is nothing I can do."

In my mind, there is *always* something one can do. But it is easy and comfortable to invent an excuse that absolves one from further action and responsibility. In the case of one's job, I might be able to understand. But in the case of one's health, this attitude leaves me dumbfounded.

So, I thought I'd list some of the more common "French Salutes" I've heard over the last two years as I've talked with people about health and wellness.

- **"We are living longer and that is why we see more chronic disease."**

This is often paired with, "This is what happens when you get old." So at what age are we "old," when chronic disease is accepted as the norm and there is really nothing more that can be done?

If this excuse were true, it would stand to reason that societies which live the longest would also have the highest incidence of heart disease, cancer, arthritis and all other diseases we associate with "old age." Not surprisingly, the opposite is true. They live the longest for the specific reason they do not suffer from these ailments.

- **"If it sounds too good to be true, it probably is."**

Imagine you are living in the 1930s. The number one cause of death is tuberculosis. Or, if you are diagnosed with venereal disease, you will simply suffer from it and probably die. Or, systemic infections will likely kill you. Then someone comes along and says, "Guess what? Moldy bread will cure all of this!" It was too good to be true, but it still was true. Sometimes the answers to the most difficult and challenging problems are also the simplest.

But, as a caveat, snake oil salesmen do exist. Let the buyer beware but also let the buyer be informed. Simply sounding too good to be true doesn't make it so.

- **"I know someone who went the 'alternative medicine' route and died anyway. So what's the point?"**

I'm guessing they also went the Western medicine route and yet they still died. I also know many terminal patients wait until they are at death's door before seeking natural approaches. Western medicine also failed them but it never seems to face the same accountability as holistic medicine.

- **"It's in my genes; I was just born that way."**

How much of it is really in one's genes; and how much has one's environment been a factor? At the grocery store I see mothers with small children and their shopping baskets are filled with processed foods, foods high in sugar and carbohydrates and extremely low in any nutritional value. If the children one day develop Type 2 diabetes, is it because their mother was also diabetic or because their mother fed them garbage? My father was one of four sons. My grandmother was diabetic as are my three uncles; yet my father never suffered from the disease. Why? Because my mother cooked and fed us healthy meals, low in sugars and carbohydrates.

Yes, I suppose some of us may be predisposed to certain illnesses but it doesn't mean we have to suffer from them. Nor does it mean there is no path to wellness.

If a mother has hypothyroidism she will likely pass it to her children. But, if the mother is properly treated for the illness before conceiving, the child will not inherit the disease.

I was born with hypothyroidism and it is likely the root cause of my heart disease. I could have simply shrugged my shoulders and said, "There is nothing I can do; I was born with this." If I had taken that attitude, I would still have the LVAD and would probably be waiting in line for a heart transplant.

- **"It's more complicated than that."**

I always want to respond to this excuse with "More complicated than what exactly? More complicated than a simple solution?" As stated above, the solution to many diseases in the early part of the twentieth century was as simple as a shot of penicillin. In the next chapter, I'll discuss the simple solution to most causes of heart disease. Preventing most forms of cancer may be as simple as taking iodine (Please read, "Iodine: Why You Need It, Why You Can't Live Without It" by Dr. David Brownstein, for a complete explanation of this statement.)

You can educate yourself and take action, or you can suffer and possibly die, from one disease or another. It's not that complicated; it's simply your choice.

Cholesterol and other Myths

"What happens when one has striven long and hard to develop a working view of the world, a seemingly useful, workable map, and then is confronted with new information suggesting that that view is wrong and the map needs to be largely redrawn? The painful effort required seems frightening, almost overwhelming. What we do more often than not, and usually unconsciously, is to ignore the new information. Often this act of ignoring is much more than passive. We may denounce the new information as false, dangerous, heretical, the work of the devil. We may actually crusade against it, and even attempt to manipulate the world so as to make it conform to our view of reality. Rather than try to change the map, an individual may try to destroy the new reality. Sadly, such a person may expend much more energy ultimately in defending an outmoded view of the world than would have been required to revise and correct it in the first place."

- M. Scott Peck, *The Road Less Traveled*

In the 1970s everyone knew that ulcers were caused by stress and dietary factors. The doctors, the government, the universities and the big pharmaceutical companies all knew this. And these same people would tell you that ulcers could not be cured. All one could do was to treat the symptoms by drinking a chalky liquid many times a day, taking antacids and avoiding spicy foods. If the ulcers began to bleed, surgery was performed.

In 1982, two Australian physicians identified the bacterium h. pylori as the true cause of ulcers and discovered it could be treated with antibiotics. They were ignored and no doubt derided for fifteen years until in 1997 when the Center for Disease Control (CDC) finally launched an education campaign to retrain doctors to treat ulcer patients with antibiotics.

And now, everyone *knows* that h. pylori, and not stress, is the true cause of ulcers. I do agree that stress, a bad diet and other factors seem to create an environment within the body which allows the h. pylori bacterium to flourish, but treating the symptoms did not cure the disease.

Imagine, science and scientific studies showed the true cause of ulcers and yet the data were basically dismissed for fifteen years.

Today, everyone knows that cholesterol causes heart disease. It is part of the American psyche. We do our best to avoid saturated (animal) fats, we eat fruits and nuts, avoid red meat, and drink non-fat milk. If our cholesterol levels rise above 200, our doctor will likely place us on a cholesterol lowering (statin) drug such as Lipitor, Crestor or Niaspan.

But what are the results of this approach? In spite of the fact that we spend over $30 billion a year on statin drugs alone plus the costs of surgery and medical devices, heart disease continues as the number one reason for death among adults. Yet if one challenges this accepted cholesterol-heart disease sacred cow, they too can expect to be derided, ignored and dismissed.

Statin drugs do lower serum cholesterol levels. From that aspect they work as advertised. Yet fifty percent of Americans who have heart attacks have cholesterol levels under 200 and the other fifty percent have levels over 200. Lowering your serum cholesterol level seems to have no statistical impact on your chances of having heart disease. You don't have to go any further than television and print ads for statin drugs to see the same information. A current television advertisement for Niaspan warns repeatedly about side effects, such as liver damage, from taking the drug. Yet, on the bottom of the screen is the following disclaimer: "Niaspan has not been shown to lower the risk of heart disease, heart attacks or stroke." It lowers serum cholesterol but it doesn't lower your risk of heart disease. (Refer to "Statin Drugs, Side Effects and the Misguided War on Cholesterol" by Dr. Duane Graveline and "Drugs That Don't Work and Natural Therapies That Do" by Dr. David Brownstein for detailed information on statins and the cholesterol/heart disease myth.)

For an excellent history of the development of the Cholesterol/Heart disease myth, read Gary Taubes' book "Good Calories. Bad Calories."

In the clinical trial for Crestor, the rate of death by heart disease in the control group (the group taking a placebo) was 2.7%. In the Crestor group, it was 2.2%. I don't see these numbers as statistically significant, yet apparently the FDA disagrees with me since they approved the drug. In other words, for one person to supposedly avoid death by heart disease, 199 additional people will receive no benefit from the drug yet will subject themselves to its devastating long-term side effects. In my opinion, that is one terrible risk/reward ratio.

In my discussions with people warning them of the dangerous side effects of statins and other drugs, one comment I have repeatedly heard is, "Yes, but not everyone experiences those side effects." That may be true, but using Crestor and Niaspan as examples, you are more likely to experience negative side effects than you are to receive benefits from the drugs.

If challenged with this information, doctors often say "It's more complicated than that." Yes, I do agree that obesity, smoking, one's diet, and lack of exercise all create an environment in the body in which heart disease can take hold; but based on the above information, why do we keep labeling cholesterol as the primary cause of heart disease? If it were true, one would think that statin drugs alone would, at a minimum, drop heart disease from the number one killer spot to at least number two or number three.

What are the long-term side effects of statin drugs? Dementia, heart failure, muscle aches, joint pain, depression and cancer and possibly Parkinson's Disease. Based on the lack of proof that Niaspan reduces the risk of heart disease and Crestor's mere one-half of one percent reduction of that same risk, why would anyone subject themselves to the potentially lethal, long-term side effects of these drugs?

Cholesterol is essential in keeping our bodies running at optimal health levels. Cholesterol delivers nutrients to every cell in our bodies.

When sick, our cholesterol levels rise as our body attempts to heal the malady. Is it any wonder as we grow older that our cholesterol levels rise to counteract the negative effects of aging? Our brains are primarily made of cholesterol. Artificially reducing the cholesterol level in our bodies increases the risk of all diseases including dementia and amnesia. Studies have shown, especially in women, that the higher their cholesterol level, the longer their life.

In 1911 famed cardiologist Paul Dudley White graduated from Harvard Medical School. Heart attacks were so rare at the time that students weren't even taught about them during their training. When Dr. White invented the electrocardiogram machine in the 1920s, he had to search for over three years to find a heart patient on whom to test the device. That is how rare heart disease was at that time. We have no way of knowing the cholesterol levels of Americans in the early 1900s, but what we do know is they were not taking statin drugs and they were not eating what we now consider to be a "heart healthy" diet. Their diets were high in animal protein, animal fats and low in sugars and non-vegetable carbohydrates.

A good friend recently visited his doctor and was told to start taking a statin drug. Based on our conversations about the dangers of cholesterol lowering drugs he told the doctor he'd rather not. The doctor insisted, but my friend could not be swayed. Finally the doctor said to him, "Ok, if you won't take the statin drug, at least do what I do and take a large dose of niacin daily." This doctor not only did not mention the niacin option up front, he also won't take the very drugs he insists on prescribing.

Probably the most famous study supposedly linking cholesterol and saturated fats to heart disease is the Framingham Study. It was conducted over a twenty-year period and included 5,000 study members. Participants were encouraged to stop smoking, lose weight, change their diets, and exercise. Of those in the study, 15% were diagnosed with heart disease in spite of their "heart healthy" lifestyles.

Dr Broda Barnes had his own theory as to the cause of heart disease and began a study patterned after Framingham. Dr. Barnes believed the root cause of most heart disease was hypothyroidism. In his study, Barnes evaluated its members for the condition based on a combination of blood tests and physical symptoms. Those showing signs were treated with natural, not synthetic, thyroid medication. The results were astonishing. By the end of Dr. Barnes' study, only two-tenths of one percent of the participants were diagnosed with heart disease.

In spite of the fact that Dr. Barnes wrote books about his findings and lectured across the country, his study has been basically ignored. Happily for me, I found a doctor who follows Barnes' advice and treats his patients accordingly.

Dr. Barnes' estimates that 40% to 50% of the population suffers from hypothyroidism at one level or another. Because of the limited testing and evaluation done by most doctors in the US regarding this disease, most go untreated. Of the cases identified, most are treated using a synthetic thyroid medication not shown to be effective. Since one of the duties of the thyroid gland is controlling the immune system, is it any wonder we see so many chronic, unexplained illnesses.

The body of evidence rejecting the cholesterol/heart disease link is extensive. I do not expect anyone to accept what I've written in this chapter at face value. You must take the time and effort and do your own research and reading. But until you, too, set aside this myth you will unlikely overcome heart disease. If you are taking statin drugs, you also significantly increase your risk of cancer, heart failure, dementia, amnesia and recently, low LDL levels have been linked to Parkinson's Disease.

For further reading I strongly suggest the following:

- "Malignant Medical Myths" by Joel M. Kaufman
- "Drugs That Don't Work And Natural Therapies That Do" by Dr. David Brownstein
- "Solved: The Riddle of Heart Attacks" by Dr. Broda Barnes

- "Statin Drugs, Side Effects and the Misguided War on Cholesterol" by Dr. Duane Graveline
- "The Untold Story of Milk" by Ron Schmid
- "Hypothyroidism, Type 2" by Dr. Mark Starr
- "Heart Disease: What Your Doctor Won't Tell You" By Dr. Rodger Murphree
- The Center for Holistic Medicine at www.drbrownstein.com

Part III

My Path

"Get busy living or get busy dying."
— The Shawshank Redemption

I have included this section for reference only. I am not suggesting you follow my path; and I am definitely not prescribing a cure for heart disease.

But, this is what I have done and what I've taken to help my body and heart heal. In many cases, I give brief explanations as to why I added a particular nutrient or food to my regimen. I say "brief" because in some cases it was added or subtracted after reading one or more books on the specific item. I choose not to go into that level of detail. Again, I hope each of you will research further about what is best for your own health.

I have broken this section, Part III, My Path, into three sub-sections:

- The first consists of the prescription medications I have taken.
- The second includes the nutrients.
- The third goes into my dietary routine and the foods that I include and those I exclude.

In the second sub-section on nutrients, I have provided brief explanations of only a few of the items. All contribute to either my general health or specifically to heart health and repair. The doses listed are those I have taken while working to heal my heart. For detailed information, I refer you to the Life Extension Foundation website (www.lef.org). Life Extension has been my principle source of supplements for the last twenty years.

For further reading about the hormones, including somatropin (HGH), testosterone and DHEA, I recommend "The Miracle of Natural Hormones" by Dr. David Brownstein.

Prescription Medications

Armour Thyroid – 90 mg daily. Armour is a natural thyroid medication made from the desiccated thyroid of a pig. I have listened to many protests by endocrinologists as to why Armour should not be taken, but I have also read all of the arguments supporting its use. I rejected prescriptions from doctors of the synthetic form of thyroid most commonly known as Synthroid. There are both alternative natural and synthetic forms available under different names.

Probably the best two resources to understand the testing and evaluation of a patient for hypothyroidism and to understand the benefits of Armour versus synthetic forms of thyroid medication are:

- "Overcoming Thyroid Disorders" by Dr. David Brownstein, and
- "Hypothyroidism: Type 2" by Dr. Mark Starr

Somatropin (Human Growth Hormone) – 30 mg daily/6x weekly. Somatropin must be kept refrigerated and is injected just under the skin in a fatty area of the body. Human growth hormone helps reverse many of the signs of aging. HGH has also been shown to improve cardiomyopathy (what I have) and congestive heart failure (CHF).

The benefits are great but the cost is high. HGH is rarely covered by insurance, but I feel it has been worth the cost for my situation. Obviously, the lower the dose, the lower the monthly cost.

Testosterone – 50 mg/2x weekly. Heart patients often have reduced levels of testosterone in their blood. This was also my case. Testosterone can be prescribed in a cream, by monthly injections or, as in my case, twice weekly injections.

Coreg (Carvedilol) – 12.5 mg/2x daily. Coreg is a beta-blocker and is often prescribed for patients with high blood pressure. Cardiologists will often also prescribe it for sufferers of cardiomyopathy as there appears to be a healing property to the drug. Following the removal of the LVAD, my goal, under the direction of my doctor, is to reduce the dose and eventually be weaned off it.

Lisinopril – 10 mg/2x daily. Lisinopril is an ace inhibitor and is also often prescribed for patients with high blood pressure. As my heart healed, it began competing with the LVAD pump. My blood pressure rose and I began experiencing severe headaches. My doctor then prescribed Lisinopril.

Amiodarone – 200 mg daily. Amiodarone is used to treat and prevent certain types of serious, life-threatening ventricular arrhythmias.

Nutrients and Supplements

Coenzyme Q10 (CoQ10) – 600 mg daily. I take CoQ10 in a softgel in the ubiquinol form. There are many benefits to taking this supplement especially for those with heart disease. Statin drugs inhibit your body's ability to convert cholesterol to this essential nutrient. If you are taking statins, you should especially consider adding CoQ10 to your daily regimen. A recent study conducted in Taiwan shows that daily doses of CoQ10 at 150mgs or higher showed significant improvement in heart disease patients.

D-Ribose – 5 grams/2x daily. I take this in a powdered form mixed with water. As with CoQ10, this is especially beneficial to patients suffering from heart disease.

L-Carnitine – 2000 mg daily.

Iodoral – (5 mg iodine/7.5 mg potassium iodide) 50 mg total daily. Iodine is an essential nutrient for all humans. It has many health benefits, including the prevention of breast and other forms of cancer. Claims of iodine poisoning from doses higher than 500 mcg are unfounded. For complete information regarding this near miracle nutrient please read, "Iodine: Why You Need It, Why You Can't Live Without It" by Dr. David Brownstein. It is important to take selenium and B-complex when taking Iodoral. Again, refer to Dr. Brownstein's book.

Selenium – 200 mcg daily.

Taurine – 2000 mg daily.

DHEA – 25 mg daily. It is not uncommon for sufferers of hypothyroidism to have hormones other than the thyroid also at reduced levels. In my case, DHEA was one of them. Like many hormones, the blood serum levels decline as we age.

Carnosine – 1000 mg daily.

Cod Liver Oil – 3 softgel capsules daily.

Niacin – 500 mg daily.

PQQ (Pyrroloquinoline Quinone) – 20 mg daily.

Calcium Citrate – **800 mg daily.** Calcium is essential for healthy bones and teeth. It should never be taken in the form of calcium carbonate, the most commonly sold form on the market, as it is poorly absorbed. Calcium should always be taken along with magnesium citrate for maximum absorption.

Magnesium Citrate – 320 mg daily.

Vitamin E – 800 IU daily

Vitamin D3 – 5,000 IU daily

B-Complex
Thiamin (B1) – 100 mg
Riboflavin (B2) – 50 mg
Niacin (B3) – 200 mg
Vitamin B6 – 75 mg
Folic Acid – 800 mcg
Vitamin B12 – 1000 mcg
Biotin – 600 mcg
Panothenic Acid – 1000 mg

Vitamin A – 10,000 IU daily

Vitamin C – 3,000 mg daily

Methylcobalamin (B12) – 5 mg daily

Zinc – 50 mg daily

High Vitamin Butter Oil – 2 capsules daily. Green Pasture X-Factor Gold

Conjugated Linoleic Acid – 1000 mg daily

Betaine HCL. This adds acid to your stomach which works to help your body properly break down and extract the nutrients from your foods. If you suffer from chronic heartburn, the problem isn't too much acid, it is not enough acid. I also try to have a glass of wine with every meal when possible.

Whey Protein Powder – 17.5 grams daily. Only take protein from whey, never soy.

Diet and Nutrition

No doubt there will be many surprises in this section for those who believe they are eating a "heart healthy" diet. Since so much of our current view of nutrition is driven by the myth that cholesterol is bad for us, is it any wonder how unhealthful our diets truly have become?

The tone and approach for my views of food and nutrition started with my mother. As a young adult she told me, "Only shop the perimeter of the supermarket. There's nothing worth eating in the center sections." Although still basically true, there is less and less worth eating around the perimeter of most major markets, as well.

There is a higher cost for many nutrient-dense foods such as raw milk or eggs from organically fed, cage-free chickens, but in comparison to the food choices of many Americans, the price is quite reasonable. A half-gallon of raw, whole milk costs about $8.50 and a dozen organic eggs, $3.50 or $12 for the shopping trip. Compare this to two breakfast meals at McDonald's for $13.00. Which is the better and healthier value and choice?

If you join the Weston A Price Foundation, they will send you a shopping guide listing different foods and the best, most nutrient-dense brands to buy. Their website is a wealth of information on all aspects of your health.

As in the section on nutrients and supplements, my explanations will be brief. I strongly recommend reading the following:

- "Nourishing Traditions" by Sally Fallon
- "Eat Fat, Lose Fat" by Mary Enig
- "Know Your Fats: The Complete Primer for Understanding the Nutrition of Fats, Oils and Cholesterol" by Mary Enig
- "The Untold Story of Milk" by Ron Schmid
- The Weston A Price Foundation website (www.westonaprice.org)

My Diet – What I Do Eat

Two eggs, lightly fried in butter, daily. The eggs are from chickens that have been organically fed and raised cage-free. The more nutritious the chicken feed, the more nutritious the eggs. It is also important that the chickens roam cage-free as they pick up additional nutrients from eating bugs and other organic material not available when caged.

One cup organic, plain, whole milk yogurt, daily. There should be only two ingredients listed on your container of yogurt: milk and culture. Check the ingredients listed on a container of yogurt from your supermarket and see how much additional and unhealthful garbage is added to such a perfect food. The brand I buy is Strauss which is also available at Trader Joe's markets under their own label as European Style. Again, only eat whole milk yogurt, never low or non-fat. If you need to add sweetener, try adding a small amount of raw, organic honey or, as I do, a small teaspoon of organic jam.

One pint whole, raw milk from pasture fed cows, daily. Yes, *raw, whole* milk; *never* low-fat or non-fat. Milk is a complete food full of protein, vitamins, minerals and enzymes. Any claims that raw and pasteurized milk are the same are completely unfounded. Several studies have been conducted where calves were separated into two groups. One group was fed raw milk and the other was fed pasteurized milk. Within one year, the pasteurized milk fed calves were either dead or faring poorly. The raw milk fed calves were thriving. Pasteurization changes the structure and nutritional value of milk. Milk that has been ultra-pasteurized at high heat has basically no nutritional value at all.

The dangers of raw milk are also greatly overstated and over-dramatized. Raw milk, if properly handled, is safer than pasteurized, homogenized milk from containment dairies.

Milk is an important food to add to your diet. For detailed information on the amazing beverage, please read, "The Untold Story of Milk" by Ron Schmid.

People who are lactose intolerant will find they can most likely drink raw milk. Raw, whole milk provides the enzymes and fats necessary for the body to properly break down and absorb its nutrients.

Butter, organic, from pasture fed cows. Like raw milk and eggs, butter packs a nutritional wallop and should be incorporated into everyone's diet.

Cheese made from raw milk. I often eat this as a snack between meals. Cheese from raw milk can often be found in specialty markets.

Red meat, organic from pasture-fed cows. I eat red meat approximately five to seven times a week. Besides eggs, red meat has probably gotten the worst, undeserved rap by the supposed "healthy diet" crowd.

Chicken, organic, free-range. I usually buy a whole chicken, roast it, then cut it up and add it to other dishes.

Organ meat. Like red meat, the organs of animals have been deemed unhealthy because of their cholesterol content, yet they are high in nutritional value. People in the southwest of France have a diet high in duck and goose liver; yet not only do they have a very low incidence of heart disease, they also are some of the most healthy and long-lived people on earth.

Vegetables, organic. As I stated in the section "My Journey" I buy a wide variety of vegetables, chop them finely and add them to almost all of the foods I cook. I also take these same chopped vegetables and naturally ferment them for use on salads. Refer to "Nourishing

Traditions" for information on fermenting vegetables and an explanation of their health benefits.

Salt, raw and organic. I buy Celtic sea salt from an online store. There are many brands of raw salt and those harvested from the Brittany coast of France are some of the best. Salt, in its raw form, is necessary for human life. Like most products, processed salt, which is what most of us use, is not healthy. Please read "Salt Your Way To Health" by Dr. David Brownstein for more information on the subject. You will also learn why lowering your salt intake does not lower your blood pressure – another common myth.

My Diet – What I Don't Eat

Soy and all soy byproducts. Soy is one of the worst possible foods you can include in your diet. Soy is what is referred to as an anti-nutrient. Instead of supplying your body with needed nutrition, it does the reverse. Nutrients are lost as your body tries to digest and process this unhealthful food. As I stated earlier, the more a food is processed, the less nutritional value it contains. Soy is one of the most processed foods on the shelf. You only need to read a description of how soy milk is made to cause you to stop drinking it for life. Soy is cheap and is the reason it is used in so many foods. Pick up almost any packaged food in the market, including salad dressings, and you will find soybean oil, soy protein, soy lecithin or some other soy byproduct in the list of ingredients. Soy protein is used by some fast food restaurants in the meats as an inexpensive extender.

If you believe soy is good for you, please read "The Whole Soy Story" by Kaayla T. Daniel.

Sugar in any form, including sugar substitutes. Sugars and other non-vegetable carbohydrates are the principle cause of heart disease, type 2 diabetes, and obesity. It is interesting that the FDA is extremely concerned about the supposed dangers of raw milk but care nothing about the population, especially children, drinking gallon after gallon of high sugar soda.

Ideally, you should use no form of sweetener, but I also know that is an almost unattainable goal for most people. If you do need something to add to your coffee or tea, use raw organic honey, or as I do, rapadura, a very raw form of cane sugar.

Fruit Juice. The reason for avoiding fruit juices is not because they are necessarily "unhealthy." Fruit juices are high in sugar, albeit natural sugars. Eating one orange may be good for you, but one glass of its juice may have been made from four or five oranges. That's a pretty big, single hit of sugar. There is a reason fruit juice is given to diabetics in insulin shock. It is a big hit of sugar that is quickly absorbed into the blood.

White flour. It's best to avoid all bread, especially if you are trying to lose or maintain your weight. Because of the fermentation process, sourdough bread is one of the better choices in this category. Whole wheat and grain breads are better than those made from white flour, but they are still carbohydrates.

Processed Foods. I see mothers in markets loading up their baskets with frozen, processed dinners for themselves and their children. To top it off, they have six packs of soda and other high-sugar drinks with which to wash it all down. If it were up to me, this would be under the heading of "child abuse." Is it any wonder that we, as a country, keep getting fatter and sicker as each year passes?

Vegetable oils. All vegetable oils, except for extra virgin olive oil, are extruded under very high heat. Heat breaks down the oil causing it to be rancid. Although it may smell fine, it is very unhealthful for your body. Also, many vegetable oils and blends are made from soybeans.

For low-heat cooking, use butter or extra virgin olive oil. For high-heat cooking, use coconut oil, duck fat, or lard.

Make your own salad dressings using extra virgin olive oil. Do not use mayonnaise, unless you make your own, because it too is usually made with soybean oil.

Anything marked low-fat, low-calorie, or diet – avoid these processed foods. Nothing good can come from them.

Deep fried foods. What type of oil is used to deep fry most foods? Soybean oil and shortening made from soybean oil. Just say no.

Toothpaste containing fluoride. No, this isn't a food, but it is important enough for me to include in this section. Fluoride has never been proven to reduce the incidence of tooth decay, yet fluoride is a poison to our bodies and is still added to most toothpastes. Our teeth do not decay because of the lack of fluoride. Our teeth decay primarily from the lack of proper nutrients and diet. I use Tom's of Maine brand toothpaste, one of which is made without fluoride.

Conclusion

I've decided to keep my conclusion brief:

1. Read and research the best path to health, for yourself and for your family.
2. Exercise, even if only a daily, brisk walk.
3. Prepare and cook your own meals using organically raised vegetables and meats.

If you don't think you have time in your busy schedule to do these things, I have to ask, why do you think you'll have time for a chronic illness, hospitalization or even death?

Choose health. Choose life.

References and Online Resources

On hypothyroidism and heart disease and the dangers of statin drugs:

Drugs that Don't Work and Natural Therapies That Do! by Dr. David Brownstein
Overcoming Thyroid Disorders by Dr. David Brownstein
Salt Your Way To Health by Dr. David Brownstein
The Miracle of Natural Hormones by Dr. David Brownstein
Hypothyroidism: Type 2 by Dr. Mark Starr
Statin Drugs, Side Effects and the Misguided War on Cholesterol by Dr. Duane Graveline
Heart Disease: What Your Doctor Won't Tell You by Dr. Rodger Murphree
Malignant Medical Myths by Joel M. Kaufman
Solved: The Riddle of Heart Attacks by Dr. Broda Barnes
The Broda Barnes Foundation at www.brodabarnes.org
The Whitaker Wellness Center at www.whitakerwellness.com

On Diet and Nutrition, nutrients:
The Untold Story of Milk by Ron Schmid
Salt Your Way To Health by Dr. David Brownstein
Good Calories. Bad Calories by Gary Taubes
Nourishing Traditions by Sally Fallon
Eat Fat, Lose Fat by Mary Enig
The Whole Soy Story by Kaayla T. Daniel
Food Is Your Best Medicine by Henry G. Bieler
Know Your Fats: The Complete Primer for Understanding the Nutrition of Fats, Oils and Cholesterol by Mary Enig
The Center for Holistic Medicine at www.drbrownstein.com
The Weston A Price Foundation at www.westonaprice.org
The Life Extension Foundation at www.lef.org

CPSIA information can be obtained at www.ICGtesting.com
Printed in the USA
LVOW040827271111

256598LV00004B/3/P